Workbook to Accompany

INTENSIVE CORONARY CARE

Fourth Edition

Jacquelyn Deal, R.N.

Robert J. Brady Co., Bowie, Maryland 20715
A Prentice-Hall Publishing and Communications Company

CONTENTS

Let's Get Acquainted

Come on in to CCU:

closed shades—
hushed voices—
flashing lights—
buzzing alarms—
Scary.
Now here's a closer view:
pleading eyes—
reaching hands—
healing hearts—
needing you—
Patients.

Do come in. Let's get to know each other. You're obviously interested in coronary care nursing, or you wouldn't be here. It really would be much nicer if we could meet over coffee or at the Coronary Care Unit desk, but at the moment let's get acquainted through the pages of this book. I'll just be myself and talk with you, and I'd love it if you would talk back to me—laugh, disagree, argue, whatever.

I'm a coronary care nurse of the 7–3, 3–11, 11–7 variety, and I'd like to introduce you to a world I love. I hope that I can help you enter this world without the usual cold hands and knocking knees, and that you'll learn to love it, too.

While I've taught coronary care classes and done inservice education, I'm not comfortable as a formal instructor. (I tend to sit on tables and discuss rather than lecture.) So I'd prefer to help you on a one-to-one basis. And that's what this book is all about. I plan, in a sense, to sit by your side (or at least be at the nurses' station) while you begin your studies in coronary care. Through these pages I'll share some of my ideas with you, ask you some questions to see if you understand the material, and try in a variety of informal ways to make your introduction to coronary care a pleasant and valuable experience.

Since we can't actually sit side by side during your training course, I had to find a common meeting ground for our discussions, and I chose to use *Intensive Coronary Care—A Manual for Nurses, Fourth Edition,* for this purpose. This wasn't a very difficult decision, since the "yellow manual" (as it is popularly called) is by far the best known book in the field, and the majority of nursing schools use it as the text for their coronary care courses. Any book that has sold nearly 800,000 copies and has been translated into four languages must have something special going for it. By going through the Manual together, we will be able to find many things to talk about.

However, *A Workbook to Accompany Intensive Coronary Care* is more than a coattail rider. It doesn't attempt to simply present the information in a different way. Instead it is meant to help you sort out the facts, apply what you learn, and test your own knowledge. Here are a few of the methods I have used in trying to make this a useful guide:

Situations: Role-plays, dialogues, and case studies are presented. These are designed to make you feel "you are there" and encourage you to exercise your judgment and knowledge. Use your imagination to project yourself into these situations: make mistakes on "my" patients; then do it right on your own. At times, I'll ask you to pretend that you're in charge of a CCU.

Questions and fill-in-the-blanks: In these pages you'll find hundreds of specific questions to test your knowledge. In many instances they follow a programmed approach leading you step by step to a conclusion. Answers are provided so that you may check yourself. In the sections where the answers are shown in the right-hand column directly across from the questions, put a 2-inch-wide strip of paper over the answer column. Read the first question, answer it in your own mind, and fill in the answer blank. Then move the strip of paper down to expose the answer. Were you right? Congratulations! Were you wrong? Well, now you know what the correct answer is. Go ahead and complete the rest of the questions in this manner.

Application: You'll also be invited to ask yourself, your doctors, and your colleagues questions, and then draw your own conclusions. Some questions are purely reflective; answer them in the context of your own situation and environment. I don't have all the answers, as you will see.

Crossword Puzzles: These are a fun way to test your knowledge. I love doing them, but making them is something else! (I'm indebted to my 12-year-old friend Holly Bayer and her mother, Mary, for helping me with these.) If crossword puzzles are a bore to you, don't fret; just answer the questions and check the results on the completed puzzle.

Word Rounds: This type of word game is quite popular among puzzle enthusiasts, and I think it can help make learning less stuffy. I'll explain how to play word rounds when we get to them. Again, if "games" don't appeal to you, use these exercises to check your knowledge by simply answering the questions.

Electrocardiographic Rhythm Strips: I've selected a series of rhythm strips taken in my own coronary unit for us to go over together. I'll tell you a little about the patients, and we'll see what you would do under the circumstances. Incidentally, don't worry about interpreting electrocardiograms. If you can master a temperature graph, you'll be able to conquer electrocardiograms.

Now that I've told you something about the contents of the *Workbook*, I should point out that you can use the book in different ways. You can choose the method that suits you best:

1. For each chapter in Dr. Meltzer's Manual, there's a corresponding chapter in the *Workbook*. You may wish to read an entire chapter in the Manual first, and then pick up the *Wookbook* so that we can go through the material in that chapter together.

2. You may prefer to start with the *Workbook* and then read the appropriate pages in the Manual as they relate to each subject being discussed. The *Workbook* clearly lists where the material can be found in the Manual.

3. You may go back and forth with the two books. Read a whole chapter in the Manual and then return to various sections as we come to them in our discussion from the *Workbook.*

4. Finally, if you're using a text other than *Intensive Coronary Care—A Manual for Nurses,* you can still put the *Workbook* to good use, both as a workbook and as a means of testing your knowledge. After all, even though the texts are different, they should cover the same fundamental material.

Before we begin, I'd like you to reassure yourself that you're not a complete stranger in foreign territory. Ask yourself the following questions and as you think about your answers, please, realize how much you already know about coronary care nursing.

1. Have I seen or cared for patients with heart attacks?
2. Can I remember how those patients felt and acted?
3. Can I remember some of the problems they had?
4. Has a family member or friend ever had angina or a heart attack?
5. Can I list some of their symptoms?
6. What else do I know about coronary heart disease?

The point is that you are not really entering an unknown world. You've already had some experience in dealing with coronary disease. In fact, you probably know a great deal about this illness. We're ready to start organizing that knowledge and building on it. You have a way to go and the aim of this book is to see that you don't get lost.

Coronary Heart Disease

ANATOMY REVIEW

Intensive Coronary Care: A Manual for Nurses, 4th edition, briefly reviews the anatomy of the heart and the circulatory system. Have you got it? To find out, do Exercise 1 now.

Exercise 1

A. Fill in the correct names of the chambers, valves, and vessels as numbered in Figure 1.1. Cover the answers at the right.

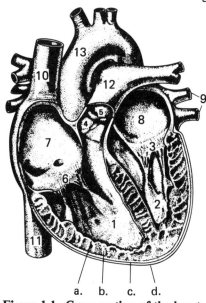

Figure 1.1. Cross section of the heart.

1. _____	right ventricle
2. _____	left ventricle
3. _____	bicuspid, or mitral, valve
4. _____	semilunar aortic valve
5. _____	semilunar pulmonary valve
6. _____	tricuspid valve
7. _____	right atria
8. _____	left atria
9. _____	pulmonary vein
10. _____	superior vena cava
11. _____	inferior vena cava
12. _____	pulmonary arteries
13. _____	aorta

B. Describe how blood circulates through the heart and major vessels. Use the appropriate numbers from Figure 1.1 for each part you list.

Venous blood returns to the heart through the _____ and the _____. It then passes through _____, _____, _____, _____, and _____ to reach the lungs. From the lungs it moves through the _____, _____, _____, _____, _____, and _____ to the body.

10, 11
7, 6, 1, 5, 12
9, 8, 3
2, 4, 13

C. Name the three layers of the heart wall as lettered in Figure 1.1.

    a. _____   endocardium

    b. _____   myocardium

    c. _____   epicardium

D. What is the membrane surrounding the heart? _____   pericardium

How did you do? If you're dissatisfied, why not dig out your old anatomy and physiology book and refresh your memory. When you are satisfied with your knowledge, go on to the next section.

CORONARY ARTERIES (*ICC, 4th ed., pp. 1-2*)

An erroneous conception held by many patients (and perhaps a few nurses as well) is that the heart muscle feeds from the blood within its chambers. Actually, the myocardium (heart muscle) receives oxygen from blood carried by the coronary arteries. If a coronary arterial branch becomes blocked, the area of heart muscle it serves is deprived of oxygen. This can cause a heart attack. In order to understand heart attacks, you must have a basic knowledge of the coronary arteries.

Exercise 2

1. There are _____ main coronary arteries that carry blood to the myocardium.   2

2. These arteries are called the _____ coronary artery and the _____ coronary artery.   left, right

3. The left coronary artery divides into two large branches: the _____ _____ _____ artery and the _____ _____ artery.   left anterior descending (LAD), left circumflex (LCA)

Let's use abbreviations from now on.

4. The term *anterior* in LAD refers to the _____ part of the heart.   front

5. Thus, the LAD serves the anterior wall of the _____.   ventricle

6. The LAD also supplies the anterior portion of the _____ _____.   interventricular septum

Stop and visualize this before continuing.

7. The other main branch of the left coronary artery is the _____ _____ _____.   left circumflex artery (LCA)

8. This branch serves the left _____ and the _____ aspect of the left _____. (See Fig. 1.1 and 1.2, *ICC,* 4th ed., pp. 1 and 2, if you're confused.)   atrium, lateral ventricle

9. The right coronary artery also arises from the _____.   aorta

10. It serves both the right _____ and the right _____.   atrium, ventricle

11. The right coronary artery comes down the (anterior/posterior) surface of the heart.   posterior

12. Thus it serves the _____ portion of the _____ ventricle.   posterior, left

13. It also serves the posterior portion of the _____ _____. (*Note:* Coronary artery patterns vary; this is the most common.)   interventricular septum

14. There (are/are not) many other small arterial branches that serve the myocardium.   are

15. The branches (do/do not) interconnect to form a network.   do

16. Each minute 250 ml of blood passes through the coronary arteries carrying oxygen to the myocardium.

    How many milliliters of blood per hour is this? _____   15,000 ml

    How many liters per hour? _____   15 liters

How many milliliters of blood per 24 hours? _____ 360,000 ml
How many liters of blood per 24 hours? _____ 360 liters
(Imagine squeezing a bulb syringe about 70 times a minute and ejecting 15 liters of
water into a sink for 1 hour. In effect, your heart does just that!)

CORONARY ATHEROSCLEROSIS (*ICC, 4th ed., pp. 2-3*)

Now you know a bit about the coronary arteries and the tremendous blood flow they
handle constantly. Next let's think about the disease process that blocks them and interferes with the passage of this 360,000 ml of blood per day to the myocardium.

Exercise 3

1. The most common disease affecting the coronary arteries is called

   _____.   atherosclerosis

2. As a result of this process the coronary arteries may become _____   narrowed
   (_____) and the blood supply to the myocardium   (obstructed)
   _____.   diminished

3. If the myocardial blood supply becomes insufficient to meet the metabolic demands of the heart, then _____ _____ _____   coronary heart disease
   (_____) exists.   (CHD)

4. Which of the following is a critical factor in CHD?
   A. The existence of atherosclerosis.
   B. The extent of arterial narrowing.   B
   C. The presence of plaque in the arteries.

5. The extent of arterial obstruction resulting in atherosclerosis is as follows:
   Grade _____ = _____ reduction of arterial lumen   1, 25
   Grade _____ = _____ reduction of arterial lumen   2, 50
   Grade _____ = _____ reduction of arterial lumen   3, 75
   Grade _____ = _____ reduction of arterial lumen   4, 100

6. Obstruction of less than _____% can usually be tolerated.   75

7. Grades _____ or _____ are considered significant obstructions. 3, 4

8. Atherosclerosis is most dangerous when the narrowing involves which main
   coronary artery? _____   Left

9. This is because it would affect circulation through the left _____   anterior
   _____ and the _____   descending,   circumflex
   arteries.

10. The left _____ _____ artery supplies blood to the   anterior descending
    anterior wall of the left and right ventricle.

11. An x-ray technique called_____ _____ can be used   coronary arteriography
    to determine the extent of coronary atherosclerosis.

12. The exact cause of coronary atherosclerosis (is/is not) known.   is not

CAUSES OF CORONARY HEART DISEASE:
RISK FACTORS (*ICC, 4th ed., pp. 3-6*)

The concept of risk factors is vitally important. Because we still don't know how to
prevent or cure coronary heart disease, we can only attempt to control these risk
factors.

To become more familiar with the dangers associated with risk factors, read some of the booklets published by the American Heart Association.* These pamphlets give you many of the facts you will need to answer the questions your patients may ask you about risk factors.

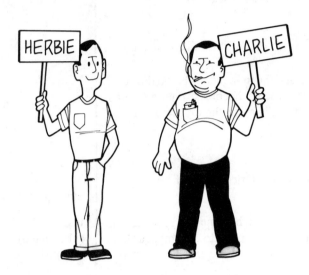

Figure 1.2.

Exercise 4

Let's compare the risk of a heart attack to two middle-aged men. Good old Herbie is normal—and, I suspect, a little blah. He has none of the risk factors mentioned on pp. 3-6 of *ICC*, 4th ed. Chubbie Charlie, on the other hand, has a few problems. He is overweight, diabetic, has high blood pressure, and smokes 2 packs of cigarettes a day.

1. What would you guess are Charlie's chances of having a heart attack before the age of 65?
   1 in _____. (Go ahead, guess.)   2, or a 50% chance

2. What about Herbie's? 1 in _____.   50, or a 2% chance

Furthermore, the American Heart Association warns people like Charlie that, if they do have a heart attack, their chances of *dying* are much greater than Herbie's because Charlie is a *smoker*.

Exercise 5

Perhaps making profiles of individuals with low- and high-risk factors would help us visualize the *importance* of risk factors. The person with low-risk factors stands a lesser chance of developing CHD, while the person with many risk factors has a greater chance of developing CHD.

For each category listed, fill in the blanks in the following table. (Use numbers for blood pressure and serum cholesterol and short, descriptive terms for the other risk factors.) One pair is filled in as an example.

---

*Two very good pamphlets are *Your Heart Has Nine Lives* and *Reduce Your Risk of a Heart Attack*.

Table 1.1. Types of Risk Factors by Degree and Category

Categories	Low Risk	High Risk
1. Sex	women	men
2. Sex and age		
3. Family history of CHD		
4. Metabolic diseases		
5. Weight		
6. Diet		
7. Serum cholesterol		
8. Triglycerides		
9. Blood pressure		
10. Cigarette smoking		
11. Activity		
12. Life-style		
13. Personality type		

Table 1.1. Answers

Categories	Low Risk	High Risk
1. Sex	women	men
2. Sex and age	women under 40	men over 50
3. Family history of CHD	none	paternal history
4. Metabolic diseases	none	especially diabetes, gout
5. Weight	normal	obese
6. Diet	low fat	high fat
7. Serum cholesterol	below 190	over 240
8. Triglycerides	below 200	above 200
9. Blood pressure	below 160/95	above 160/95
10. Cigarette smoking	nonsmoker	smoker
11. Activity	active	sedentary
12. Life-style	nonstressful	stressful
13. Personality type	Type B	Type A

LDL, VLDL, HDL, AND CHD (*ICC, 4th ed., p. 4*)

Exercise 6

From now on we'll abbreviate coronary heart disease as CHD. (Nurses don't mind abbreviations; it's the doctor's handwriting that we can't stand!) Lest mass confusion overcome us, let's spend a few minutes with all the initials used above.

1. Specifically, Dr. Meltzer et al. talk about two serum lipids, _____ and _____.

   cholesterol
   triglycerides

2. These two lipids are (soluble/insoluble) in plasma.

   insoluble

3. However, when combined with protein "carriers," they become _____ _____, which are soluble.

   lipoproteins

4. There are three main classes of lipoprotein (Initials, please). _____ _____ _____.

   LDL, VLDL, HDL

5. One at a time now: VLDL stands for _____ _____-_____ _____.

   very low-density lipoproteins

6. LDL stands for _____-_____ _____.

   low-density lipoproteins

7. HLD stands for _____-_____ _____.

   high-density lipoproteins

8. _____ carries more of the cholesterol in the blood.

   LDL

9. _____ carries more of the triglycerides in the blood.

   VLDL

10. Serum cholesterol and triglyceride levels (are/are not) necessarily related. | are not

11. Now, let's oversimplify and classify these three as "good guys" or "bad guys." The "good guy" that seems to *protect* against CHD is _____. | HDL

12. High levels of LDL (increase/decrease) the risk of CHD. | increase

This diagram should help you remember.

$$\uparrow LDL = \uparrow CHD$$
$$\uparrow VLDL = \uparrow CHD$$
$$\uparrow HDL = \downarrow CHD$$

CLASSIFICATION OF CORONARY HEART DISEASE (*ICC, 4th ed., pp. 6-11*)

Exercise 7

To help you fix the classification of CHD firmly in your mind, complete the following statements.

1. CHD is caused by obstruction in the coronary _____. | arteries

2. Minimal obstruction may not decrease the blood supply to the _____. | myocardium

3. Minimal obstruction is unlikely to produce symptoms and may be discovered only after an _____. | autopsy

4. Coronary arteries may be grossly obstructed but still not produce any _____. | symptoms

5. This is because the oxygen needs of the myocardium have been supplied by _____ circulation. | collateral

6. Coronary atherosclerosis (is/is not) synonymous with CHD. | is not

7. Inadequate blood supply to the myocardium results in a lack of _____ for the cardiac cells. | oxygen

8. Insufficient oxygenation is called _____. | ischemia

9. Myocardial ischemia causes chest pain known as _____ _____. | angina pectoris

10. Angina pectoris is classified as a form of _____ CHD. | symptomatic

11. In order of severity, the three clinical patterns of CHD are: *angina pectoris,* _____ _____ _____, (also known as _____ angina), and _____ _____ _____ _____. | intermediate coronary syndrome, unstable, acute myocardial infarction

ANGINA PECTORIS (*ICC, 4th ed., pp. 6*)

Angina pectoris is one of the most important symptoms of CHD. Note how carefully the chest pain pattern is described in *ICC,* 4th ed. Because you will have to decide whether a patient is experiencing angina, you will need a clear understanding of the clinical picture.

Exercise 8

1. Angina is characterized by its _____ (or precordial) location. | substernal

2. It frequently radiates to any of several sites, including the arms, _____, _____, _____, _____ _____. | neck jaw, teeth, upper back

3. The pain (is/is not) relieved by changes in breathing or position. | is not

4. The pain is usually described as a _____ or a _____. | pressure, tightness

5. The pain often begins during _____ _____. | physical exertion

6

6. It usually _____ as soon as activity ceases.   stops

7. Thus, it is termed _____ of _____.   angina, effort

8. It is possible for _____ as well as physical stress to induce angina.   emotional

9. Any stress that increases the heart_____ or blood_____ may induce angina.   rate, pressure

10. Angina generally lasts _____ minutes.   1-5

11. It is almost always relieved by _____.   nitroglycerin

12. Nitroglycerin _____ the coronary arteries.   dilates

13. This (increases/decreases) the blood and oxygen supply to the myocardium.   increases

14. The most common side effect of nitroglycerin is _____.   headache

15. If nitroglycerin does not relieve the pain, you should suspect the pain (is/is not) due to angina of effort.   is not

Exercise 9

1. In diagnosis of angina pectoris the most important thing is _____ _____.   patient's history

2. If you are questioning a patient about a chest pain episode, there are four areas of importance: _____, _____, _____, and _____.   location (central), duration (brief), quality (oppressive), relation to effort

3. Stress tests may be used to induce ECG evidence of myocardial _____. (If you haven't observed one, make arrangements to do so.)   ischemia

4. Chest pain during a stress test (is/is not) defined as a positive result.   is not

5. Positive stress tests require _____ _____.   ECG changes

6. One of the nuclear scanning techniques used in diagnosis of CHD is _____ _____.   radio-nuclide angiography

7. During exercise testing, muscle areas with reduced blood flow contract (normally/abnormally).   abnormally

8. An IV injection of a _____ _____ is given during the peak exercise period.   radioactive isotope

9. The nuclear camera will record abnormal ventricular contractions in _____ areas.   ischemic

10. The most definitive method of diagnosis is _____ _____.   coronary arteriography

11. This involves inserting a catheter through a peripheral artery into the root of the _____ and injecting radiopaque dye into the _____ _____ _____.   aorta, two coronary arteries

12. List three things coronary arteriography can show: _____, _____, and _____ _____.   number of vessels involved, extent of involvement, degree of collateral circulation

13. Two "invasive" diagnostic studies are _____ _____ and _____.   cardiac catheterization ventriculography

14. In cardiac catheterization, catheters are run into the heart _____ and the great _____.   chambers vessels

15. Measurements are then made of the oxygen _____ and _____ in these areas.   pressure, concentration

16. In ventriculography, a radiopaque dye is inserted through a catheter placed in the _____ _____ .   left ventricle

17. The "motion pictures" resulting are (more/less) precise than radionuclide pictures.   more

STABLE AND VARIANT ANGINA PECTORIS
(*ICC, 4th ed., pp. 8-9*)

I'll bet you knew that angina pectoris couldn't be so "stable" and simple. You were right! For years doctors have been plagued by patients with "variant" symptoms: patients who refused to conform to nice, clinical patterns of angina, yet who obviously had sick hearts. So now we have a classification for them: variant angina pectoris.

Exercise 10

To refine your knowledge about stable and variant angina, place an S (stable) or a V (variant) in front of the most appropriate statements below.

_____ 1. No pain or ECG evidence during exercise testing	1.	V
_____ 2. Fixed narrowing of arteries	2.	S
_____ 3. Also known as "classic" angina	3.	S
_____ 4. May be relieved by calcium antagonists	4.	S
_____ 5. Effectively relieved by calcium antagonists	5.	V
_____ 6. Relieved by rest	6.	S
_____ 7. Caused by coronary artery spasm	7.	V
_____ 8. Relieved with nitroglycerin	8.	S
_____ 9. Pain at rest	9.	V
_____ 10. Cyclic pain pattern	10.	V
_____ 11. Induced by physical activity	11.	S
_____ 12. Induced by emotional stress	12.	S
_____ 13. Also known as Prinzmetal's angina	13.	V
_____ 14. Often 75% narrowing of 2 or 3 arteries	14.	S

INTERMEDIATE CORONARY SYNDROME AND MYOCARDIAL INFARCTION (*IC, 4th ed., pp. 9-12*)

As you now realize, angina pectoris is only a symptom of CHD. It is a warning that the heart isn't getting all the blood it needs at that moment. Changes in the circulatory condition and patterns of the syndrome result in a progression of severity: stable or variant; then unstable; and finally the most ominous, acute myocardial infarction. Picture this progression by using your imagination. You could relate the patterns to horses: "stable," predictable ones or the "variantly" behaving, confusing ones; then the "unstable," more dangerous ones; and finally, the "acute" situation, the rider unseated, writhing on the ground. Form your own pictures to remember these terms because you're about ready to meet more new terms.

Exercise 11

ICC, 4th ed., p. 9, lists seven names for the condition you're now learning about. Find the terms used in your area and remember those. For our purposes, we'll use *unstable angina* for the *intermediate coronary syndrome*.

1. Unstable angina ranks in severity intermediate (or between) _____ _____ _____ and ____ _____ _____ _____.

    stable angina pectoris, acute myocardial infarction

2. A common feature of unstable angina is clinical (stability/instability).

    instability

3. Unstable angina pain usually lasts (1 to 5/5 to 10/10 to 20) minutes.

    10 to 20

4. Unstable angina occurs (less often/more often), can be induced by (less/greater) exertion, and (often/seldom) occurs at rest.

    more often, less often

5. Nitroglycerin's effect on unstable angina is _____.

    incomplete or none

6. ECG commonly shows signs of _____.

    ischemia

7. ECG (does/does not) show signs of acute myocardial infarction.

    does not

8. Unstable angina is (more/less) severe than stable angina.

    more

9. The immediate forerunner of acute myocardial infarction is _____ _____.

    unstable angina

MYOCARDIAL INFARCTION (*ICC, 4th ed., pp. 9-11*)

Exercise 12

Now let's use your knowledge of the coronary arterial anatomy to see what happens in a myocardial infarction (MI).

1. As you know, insufficient oxygenation of tissues is called _____.

    ischemia

2. If ischemia is severe or prolonged, tissue _____ may occur.

    destruction

3. This is called _____.

    necrosis

4. Necrotic muscle is also called _____ muscle.

    infarcted

5. A myocardial infarction means a local area of heart muscle is _____ or _____.

    dead infarcted

6. What your patient calls a heart attack, you call a _____ _____.

    myocardial infarction

7. You usually abbreviate that to _____.

    MI

8. Nearly all MIs are due to _____ _____.

    coronary atherosclerosis

9. The event producing an acute MI may be called a coronary _____ or coronary _____.

    thrombosis occlusion

10. In actual practice, the terms *myocardial infarction, heart attack,* and *coronary* are used interchangeably. (True/False)

    True

11. A coronary artery may be blocked if a _____ develops on the rough atherosclerotic plaques.

    clot

12. A coronary artery may be blocked if bleeding occurs under the plaques. That's called _____ _____.

    subintimal hemorrhage

13. Or a piece of plaque may _____ _____ and swim away to block a small artery.

    break off

14. Autopsies have shown MIs (can/cannot) occur without clots or complete arterial obstruction.

    can

15. Two possible explanations for Question 14 are: _____ _____ _____ _____ _____ _____.

    Sudden intense oxygen demand (due to exercise or stress) that the arteries can't supply or coronary arterial spasm complicating an existing coronary artery disease.

16. Blockage of the (right/left) coronary artery is usually more serious.

    left

17. The left coronary artery divides into 2 main branches, the _____ and the _____. — LAD / LCA

18. They primarily serve the (anterior/posterior) portion of the left heart. — anterior

19. Thus, occlusion of the left coronary artery is likely to cause (anterior/posterior) MI. — anterior

20. The right coronary artery travels down the back of the heart and supplies the (inferior/superior) portion of the left ventricle. — inferior

21. The inferior part of the heart is also called the _____ portion. — diaphragmatic

22. Occlusion of the right coronary artery is likely to cause an _____ MI. — inferior (or diaphragmatic)

23. If an infarction involves the anterior wall of the left ventricle and the anterior portion of the interventricular septum, the infarction would be termed an _____ MI. — anteroseptal

24. In this case, the occluded coronary artery is the _____. — LAD

25. An infarction involving the anterior and lateral aspects of the left ventricle would be termed an _____ MI. — anterolateral

26. An infarction involving the inferior and lateral walls of the left ventricle is termed an _____ MI. — inferiolateral

27. An infarction of only the right ventricle (is/is not) rare. — is

28. The extent of an infarction depends on the _____ of the artery obstructed and the degree of _____ _____ available. — size / collateral circulation

29. If an area of infarction extends clear through the ventricular wall, it is a _____ MI. — transmural

30. An infarction that does not extend through the full thickness of the ventricular wall is termed nontransmural or _____ or _____. — intramural, subendocardial

Exercise 13

Label Zones I, II, and III on the infarcted area in Figure 1.3 (*See also ICC,* 4th ed., p. 12).

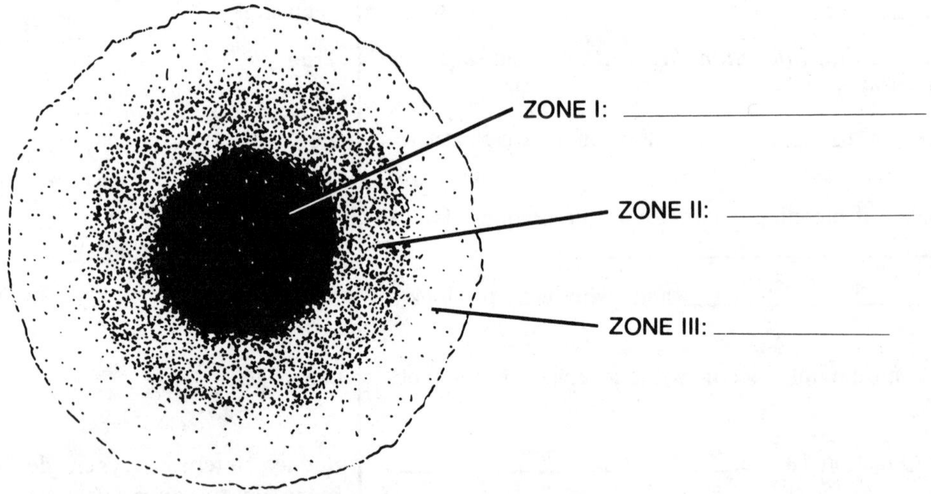

ZONE I: _____

ZONE II: _____

ZONE III: _____

Zone I: Infarction
Zone II: Injury
Zone III: Ischemia

Figure 1.3. Three zones of tissue damage associated with acute myocardial infarction.

1. Zone I is (temporarily/permanently) damaged. — permanently

2. Zone II may recover if adequate _____ is restored. — circulation

3. Zone III (often/rarely) recovers. — often

TERMINOLOGY REVIEW (*ICC, 4th ed., Chapter 1*)

You may have learned some new terms or relearned some old ones in this chapter. You can test yourself by matching terms and definitions in the following exercise. If you'd like to have a little fun with your knowledge, find about 20 buttons or pennies and play Bingo on the card following the matching test.

Exercise 14

Place the correct definition number in front of each term. Use each number only once. To play Bingo with this exercise, use the Bingo sheet that follows this test.

Definitions	Terms	
1. provide blood to nourish the heart muscle	_____ angina	11
2. muscle layer of the heart	_____ atherosclerosis	3
3. narrowing of arteries due to fatty deposits	_____ collateral circulation	10
4. fatty deposits	_____ coronary arteries	1
5. inner lining of arteries	_____ coronary heart disease	6
6. conditions occurring when blood supply to myocardium is insufficient	_____ intermediate coronary syndrome	17
7. behind the sternum		
8. observable	_____ coronary occlusion	22, 21
9. cardiac output	_____ coronary thrombosis	21, 22
10. additional secondary blood supply	_____ heart attack	23
11. chest pain due to myocardial ischemia	_____ intima	5
12. little or no activity	_____ ischemia	16
13. seemingly contradictory	_____ myocardium	2
14. gives relief from angina	_____ necrosis	20
15. underneath the lining of an artery	_____ overt	8
16. resulting from lack of oxygen		
17. unstable angina	_____ preinfarction angina	18
18. coronary insufficiency	_____ plaques	4
19. outer layer	_____ subintimal	15
20. local death of cells	_____ substernal	7
21. heart attack		
22. a "coronary"		
23. myocardial infarction		
24. under the tongue		
25. opening		

In the preceding exercise there are 18 terms and 25 definitions.

1. After you pick the definition for each term, cover the definition numbers on the Bingo card with a penny or button.

2. If you've done them correctly, the 18th definition should give you a double bingo—5 numbers covered horizontally and 5 numbers covered vertically.

1	9	5	16	8
11	14	18	23	19
13	21	25	2	12
4	17	22	20	24
3	15	6	7	10

Figure 1.4.

THE HEART OF THE MATTER (*ICC, 4th ed., Chapter 1*)

Exercise 15

1. Label the 3 coronary arteries in Figure 1.5.

1. right coronary artery
2. left circumflex artery
3. left anterior descending artery

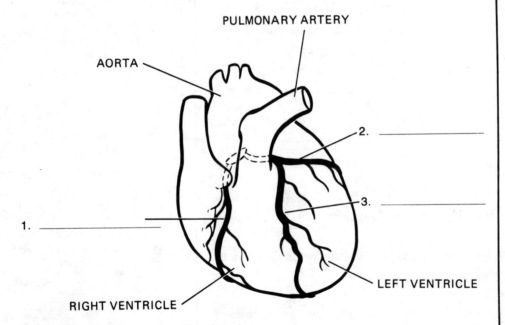

Figure 1.5. The coronary arteries of the heart.

Check your answers before continuing. Use Figure 1.5 to help you with the next questions.

2. Come on in and join the gang at Myoville General Hospital. We have three rather colorful patients with coronary heart disease. Let's see if we can visualize what has happened to the coronary arteries.

PATIENT 1: MR. T. BROWN

Draw a blood clot obstructing the coronary artery where the line for artery 1 touches the artery on Figure 1.5. Coronary arteriography demonstrates an obstruction at this point.

1. From the coronary arteriographic findings, you conclude that the _____ _____ artery is obstructed.

    right coronary

2. This means that the _____ _____ and _____ _____ may be deprived of an adequate blood supply.

    right atrium, right ventricle

3. Far more important, obstruction of the right coronary artery affects the inferior section of the _____ _____.

    left ventricle

4. It also affects the posterior portion of the _____ septum.

    interventricular

5. The obstruction of Mr. Brown's right coronary artery involves mainly the (superior/inferior) portion of his heart.

    inferior

6. The inferior portion of the heart lies near what anatomical landmark? _____.

    diaphragm

7. Therefore, the ECG diagnosis of Mr. Brown's infarction will be classified as _____ or _____.

    inferior, diaphragmatic

PATIENT 2: MR. FORREST GREEN

Draw an obstruction of the coronary artery where the line for artery 2 touches the artery on Figure 1.5

1. Mr. Green's coronary arteriogram shows that the _____ _____ artery is obstructed.

    left circumflex

2. This artery provides blood to the left_____ and the lateral aspect of the left _____.

    atrium
    ventricle

3. Mr. Green's ECG reveals changes in the_____ wall of the left ventricle.

    lateral

PATIENT 3: MRS. MISTY BLUE

Draw a plaque obstructing the coronary artery where the line for artery 3 meets the artery on Figure 1.5.

1. Mrs. Blue's coronary arteriogram shows that the _____ _____ _____ artery is obstructed.

    left anterior descending

2. This artery services the (anterior/posterior) wall of the _____ _____.

    anterior, left ventricle

3. It also serves the (anterior/posterior) portion of the _____ septum.

    anterior, interventricular

4. If Mrs. Blue's infarction involves the anterior portion of the left ventricle and the interventricular septum, it is termed an _____.

    anteroseptal

5. An obstruction of the left coronary artery *before* its bifurcation would deprive the (anterior/posterior) portion of the _____ _____, the anterior portion of the _____ _____, and also the _____ aspect of the left ventricle.

    anterior, left ventricle
    interventricular septum
    lateral

6. This could cause an extensive _____ MI.

    anterior

7. Read some of the ECGs of patients with MI. How many of these diagnostic terms can you find?

    Probably all

8. Doesn't it make you feel good to know what they mean?

    I hope so!

Now let's try a few review questions on coronary heart disease. By the time you finish these, you should have a much better understanding of this subject than you did when you started!

1. Unstable angina is (more/less) dangerous than stable angina and the patient is probably (closer to/farther from) experiencing an MI.

   more
   closer to

2. For atherosclerosis to be termed "significant" in terms of degree of obstruction, it involves at least a _____% reduction of the arterial lumen.

   75

3. This is termed Grade _____ or _____ atherosclerosis.

   3, 4

4. Generally, infarctions from the left coronary artery are (anterior/posterior).

   anterior

5. Infarctions from the right coronary artery are (superior/inferior).

   inferior

6. The (right/left) ventricle is less often infarcted.

   right

7. The areas surrounding an MI shortly after its occurrence:

   Zone I   = _____
   Zone II = _____
   Zone III = _____

   necrotic
   injured
   ischemic

2

Acute Myocardial Infarction

HISTORY AND SYMPTOMS OF ACUTE MYOCARDIAL INFARCTION (*ICC, 4th ed., p. 13*)

Mr. A is brought to the Emergency Room at 3 A.M. He is gray-faced, obviously in pain, and gasping for breath.

Nurse: What seems to be the problem?
Mr. A: This pain—I woke up with it. I feel like I'm gonna die.
Nurse: Can you tell me what the pain feels like?
Mr. A: Like a truck sitting on my chest.
Nurse: Exactly where does it hurt?
Mr. A: (*Strikes midchest with clenched fist.*) Here and all across. It's strange; my left elbow hurts, and my jaw, too.
Nurse: Has the pain eased up any since it began?
Mr. A: No, it just won't go away. I tried Alka-Seltzer and then a little whiskey— nothing helps.
Nurse: When the pain began, did you sweat?
Mr. A: My pajamas were soaked.
Nurse: Were you sick at your stomach?
Mr. A: Was I? I vomited twice already. I knew I shouldn't have eaten both lasagna and spaghetti last night.
Nurse: When did you get short of breath?
Mr. A: Right after the pain began. I couldn't get my breath.

Mrs. B comes to the Emergency Room an hour later. She is doubled up with pain, white-faced, dyspneic, and obviously frightened.

Nurse: You seem to be in pain.
Mrs. B: Oh, my chest . . .
Nurse: What is the pain like?
Mrs. B: It's like a knife—a sharp pain—it stabs here (*indicates left side of chest with one finger*).
Nurse: Is the pain continuous?

15

Mrs. B: No. It comes and goes.

 Nurse: How about breathing?

Mrs. B: I don't dare take a deep breath; it makes the pain worse.

 Nurse: Did the pain start all at once?

Mrs. B: It began gradually, but it's gotten worse.

 Nurse: Have you vomited or been nauseated?

Mrs. B: I keep belching all the time. Have I had a heart attack?

Exercise 1

Let's analyze the history and symptoms of these patients by means of a series of questions. Then read the discussion that follows.

1. Is there good reason to suspect from the history that Mr. A. has had a myocardial infarction? (Yes/No)

> Yes, the symptoms Mr. A. describes should certainly make you suspect an acute myocardial infarction.

2. What about Mrs. B? (Yes/No)

> No, Mrs. B.'s history is not suggestive of myocardial infarction.

3. What is the most important symptom in Mr. A.'s history to suggest acute myocardial infarction?

> The most important symptom is severe substernal pain which persists. This symptom alone should make you suspicious. Be aware that people interpret "pain" differently. I'm reminded of a lady who insisted, "I had absolutely no pain with my heart attack. It just felt like an elephant was sitting on my chest." Now, to me, that's pain!

4. What other symptoms of his further this suspicion?

> Pain to elbow and jaw, sweating, nausea and vomiting, shortness of breath.

5. Is the localized, knifelike pain Mrs. B. experienced characteristic of acute myocardial infarction? (Yes/No)

> No

6. What about the relationship of Mrs. B.'s chest pain to breathing? Is this a common story? (Yes/No)

> No, pain on breathing isn't a common complaint with AMI.

7. How important do you think it is for a nurse to be able to recognize acute myocardial infarction? (Very/Not very)

> Very important. Your ability to recognize the symptoms of an MI, whether in a postoperative or emergency room patient, or in your friends or family, may save a life.

CLINICAL COURSE OF MYOCARDIAL INFARCTION (*ICC, 4th ed., p. 14*)

What happens to a patient right after a heart attack? According to *ICC*, 4th ed., the clinical course is basically determined by 1) the size or extent of the infarction (transmural vs. nontransmural) and 2) the degree of collateral circulation. Good collateral circulation means that enough blood can be diverted through small, auxiliary vessels to supply the area of injured myocardium. In other words, if your large garden sprinkler plugs up, you can still save your lettuce and radishes with several smaller sprinkers. If the infarcted area is small and collateral circulation is adequate, the clinical course is likely to be good. However, if the infarction is extensive, or if enough blood cannot be brought to the injured myocardium, the prognosis if likely to be poor.

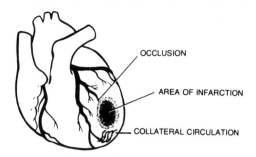

Figure 2.1A

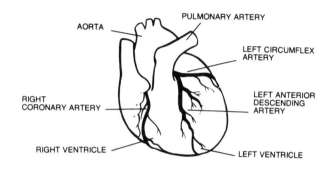

Figure 2.1B

Exercise 2

1. Do all patients with acute MI develop complications? (Yes/No)

   No

2. Can you be certain that a patient with a small infarction won't develop complications? (Yes/No)

   No

3. If a patient has a large infarction, can you be certain that complications will develop? (Yes/No)

   No

4. In other words, complications can develop in _____ patient at _____ time!

   any, any (*never forget this*)

5. Without sufficient oxygen your heart won't pump effectively. So decreased oxygenation leads to decreased _____.

   pumping

6. Decreased pumping can lead to _____ _____.

   heart failure

7. When the left ventricle is severely injured and can't pump out enough blood to meet the body's needs, vital organs such as the _____ and _____ are deprived of adequate blood and oxygen.

   brain, kidneys

8. As a result, the blood pressure _____.

   falls

9. Urinary output _____.

   decreases

10. The skin becomes _____ and _____.

    cold, clammy

11. The failing heart struggles to compensate, so it pumps _____.

    faster

12. The pulse rate (increases/decreases).

    increases

13. Questions 7-12 describe what condition? _____ _____.

    cardiogenic shock

14. Impaired oxygenation can also upset the _____ and _____ of the heartbeat.

    rate, rhythm

15. This produces _____.

    arrhythmias

16. Arrhythmias can cause _____ death.

    sudden

17. Arrhythmias can occur at _____ time in _____ patient.

    any, any

17

COMPLICATIONS OF AN MI (*ICC, 4th ed., pp. 14-15*)

Always remember—death from myocardial infarction is the result of complications. This section is just a brief overview of the 5 main complications of MI. Go through these complications one at a time. We'll be talking about them all through the book.

Exercise 3

COMPLICATION 1: ARRHYTHMIAS

1. Probably 90% of your MI patients will develop _____.

   arrhythmias

2. Arrhythmias are disturbances in _____, _____, or _____.

   rate, rhythm, conduction

3. Arrhythmias can cause sudden _____.

   death

4. Or they can reduce the _____ efficiency of the heart.

   pumping

5. _____ _____ is the arrhythmia that is the most common cause of sudden death.

   Ventricular fibrillation

COMPLICATION 2: ACUTE LEFT VENTRICULAR FAILURE

1. About 60% of your MI patients will have some clinical signs of _____ _____.

   heart
   failure

2. Heart failure occurs when the heart's _____ ability is reduced.

   pumping or contractile

3. Heart failure may develop _____ or _____.

   gradually, suddenly

4. Sudden left ventricular failure is called _____ _____.

   acute pulmonary edema

COMPLICATION 3: CARDIOGENIC SHOCK

1. Cardiogenic shock is less common than arrhythmias or heart failure, but it is more _____.

   serious

2. At least 80 to 90% of patients who develop cardiogenic shock will _____.

   die

3. Cardiogenic shock occurs when there is not enough circulation to provide adequate _____ for vital organs and tissues.

   oxygen

4. Are cardiogenic shock and heart failure identical? (Yes/No)

   No

5. Are you confused? (Yes/No)

   Probably! (If so, don't worry, we'll straighten this out in Chapter 7.)

COMPLICATION 4: THROMBOEMBOLISM

1. Blood clots may form on the inner wall of the _____ _____ after an MI.

   left ventricle

2. If these clots break loose, where would the circulation carry them? _____ _____ of the _____, _____, and _____.

   To arteries, brain, abdomen limbs

3. If a blood clot blocks an artery to the brain, the symptoms would suggest a _____.

   stroke

4. If a blood clot forms in the deep veins of the legs, the circulation would carry it through the right side of the heart to the _____.

   lungs

18

5. There, it would probably block a pulmonary artery and cause a _____ _____ or _____.

pulmonary embolism, infarction

6. Embolic complications are (common/uncommon).

uncommon

COMPLICATION 5: RUPTURE OF THE LEFT VENTRICLE

1. Rupture of the left ventricle is (common/uncommon).

uncommon

2. It occurs when a _____ area in the left ventricle _____ ruptures.

necrotic, wall

3. Blood leaves the left ventricle and fills the _____ _____.

pericardial sac

4. This results in external _____ or _____ of the heart.

compression, squeezing

5. This compression of the heart by blood in the pericardial sac is called _____ _____.

cardiac tamponade

6. Ventricular rupture is most likely to occur within the first _____ to _____ days of hospitalization.

7, 10

DIAGNOSIS OF MYOCARDIAL INFARCTION (*ICC, 4th ed., pp. 15-18*)

Many patients are admitted to a CCU. Let's see if we can go through the steps the doctors take to prove a diagnosis of MI.

Exercise 4: History and Electrocardiogram

1. The patient was admitted to the CCU because his or her _____ was indicative of myocardial infarction.

history

2. The doctor must determine if the _____ shows definite changes of an MI.

ECG

3. Lab tests will show if the _____ are elevated.

enzymes

4. A definitive diagnosis of MI cannot be made unless there are specific _____ changes.

ECG

Exercise 5: Enzyme Studies

1. Which enzyme rises first and returns to normal first after an acute MI? _____

CPK

2. Which enzyme rises next and returns to normal next? _____

SGOT

3. Which enzyme is the slowpoke? _____

LDH

4. Very high enzyme levels usually (are/are not) indicative of extensive myocardial damage.

are

To remember this order, drop the S off SGOT (it stands for serum anyway) and then put the enzymes in alphabetical order: CPK, GOT, LDH. Watching these lab reports on your cardiac patients is fascinating. Sometimes the enzymes reach frighteningly high levels (which usually means extensive myocardial damage), and then you wish you could pack your patient's heart in cotton balls to protect it.

Exercise 6:

CPK—THE EARLY BIRD

1. CPK is released after damage to the heart muscle, _____ muscles, or _____ _____.

skeletal
the brain

2. Thus CPK elevations may occur after an MI, or a fracture with _____ injury, or a _____ with brain damage.

muscle
stroke

19

3. _____ medication given to a patient may cause a slight elevation of CPK.

                    Intramuscular (IM)

4. An isoenzyme of CPK specific for myocardial necrosis is called _____.

                    CPK—MB

5. CPK rises almost immediately, within _____ to _____ hours after an MI.

                    2, 6

6. It usually peaks within _____ hours.

                    24

7. CPK levels often elevate to a greater extent than the other enzymes. (True/False)

                    True

SGOT—THE SECOND RISER

1. While CPK usually elevates within 2 to 6 hours after an MI, it takes SGOT about _____ hours to begin rising.

                    8

2. CPK peaks in 24 hours; SGOT peaks between _____ and _____ hours.

                    24, 48

3. SGOT usually returns to normal after _____ to _____ days.

                    3, 4

4. SGOT also increases in noncardiac-related diseases, particularly _____ disease.

                    liver

LDH—THE SLOWPOKE

1. LDH doesn't usually peak until the _____ to _____ day after an MI.

                    2nd, 3rd

2. LDH usually returns to normal about the _____ or _____ day after an MI.

                    5th, 6th

3. Elevation of LDH (is/is not) a definite sign of an MI.

                    is not

Exercise 7: Radionuclide Imaging

1. If other diagnostic evidence is missing or misleading, radionuclide imaging (can/cannot) be used to help diagnose an MI.

                    can

2. Two basic forms of radionuclide imaging are "_____ spot" and "_____ spot" imaging.

                    hot, cold

3. "Hot spot" imaging uses _____ 99m pyrophosphate.

                    technicium

4. Necrotic myocardium shows a (greater/lesser) uptake of the IV technicium.

                    greater

5. This increased radioactivity shows up as a _____.

                    "hot spot"

6. "Hot spot" imaging is more reliable for (transmural/nontransmural) infarctions.

                    transmural

7. "Cold spot" imaging uses _____-201.

                    thallium

8. Necrotic myocardium shows (no/a greater) uptake of thallium-201.

                    no

9. Thus, a void or "(cold/hot) spot" shows the area of necrosis.

                    cold

10. A new infarct (can/cannot) be differentiated from an old infarct with thallium.

                    cannot

11. Thallium can be used with _____ _____ to help diagnose the ischemia of angina and unstable angina.

                    exercise testing

PHYSICAL EXAMINATION *(ICC, 4th ed., pp. 18-19)*

    One of the most important parts of physical examination involves no more than just looking and talking to a patient. Observation tells you a lot. Every time you walk into a patient's room you are, in a sense, examining the patient. Use all your senses to become the best observer possible.

Exercise 8

Make a list of the important questions you might ask yourself about your next patient to be admitted to Myoville General Hospital's CCU. Then complete it with my list that follows:

_____

_____

_____

_____

_____

_____

_____

_____

_____

_____

Was patient in pain?

Was patient frightened?

Was patient short of breath?

Was he propped up in bed or could he lie flat?

Was the skin dry or clammy?

Was the skin cold or warm?

What about color? Pale, or gray, or ashen?

Did patient vomit or complain of nausea?

Was patient restless?

Was patient confused?

Was the heartbeat fast, slow, regular or irregular?

Was the BP normal?

THE ACUTE PHASE OF MI (*ICC, 4th ed., p. 19*)

Let's recap. The doctor has admitted the patient to the CCU because of suspected myocardial infarction. The history, ECG, and enzymes all say: MI. What can you expect now? Suppose we take a look at 3 patients who illustrate the "3 broad patterns" described in *ICC, 4th ed.*

1. Mrs. Glutton is a collage of risk factors. But after her pain subsides, she becomes a pain: she complains loudly about the CCU diet (low cholesterol, low calorie, low sodium), she's dying for a cigarette, she misses her favorite TV soap opera. Thankfully, she recovers uneventfully and goes home. Lucky? Or just a small infarct with good collateral circulation?

2. Mr. Thirty-nine is so young. No one can really believe he's had an MI, not even with all the diagnostic evidence that exists. He's had occasional arrhythmias, but he seems to be doing so well you just can't take them seriously. You're chatting with him one afternoon with your back to the monitor, and he's telling you a joke—but he never makes it to the punch line. Ventricular fibrillation stops him. Does he die? What do you think?

3. Mr. Hectic is so cold and clammy on admission that you wonder if he came by refrigerated van rather than by ambulance. You breathe a prayer and stick an IV needle into a vein that's hardly even there. From then on you fight; the next day, you're almost certain Mr. Hectic won't be there. And you're right.

Remember these are only general patterns of the course after an MI. Next time, Mrs. Glutton may be a number 3, and the young, strong thirty-niner may be a number 1. But don't count on it.

Exercise 9

Keep a mental scorecard on the next patients you see with acute MI. Into which category do they fall?

OTHER ASPECTS OF THE
ACUTE PHASE (*ICC, 4th ed., p. 20*)

You've just started on the night shift at Myoville General Hospital. It's Deal's axiom that anything that can go wrong, will go wrong—at night—especially if you don't have a house doctor. Myoville doesn't have a house doctor (how did you guess?).

During your first week on night duty, your cardiac patients exhibit the 22 responses listed below. Some of these responses you expect and you won't wake up the doctor because of them. Other responses you feel are unexpected and you'd probably call the doctor.

Exercise 10

Mark the expected ones with an *E* and the unexpected ones with a *U*.

_____	1. Drooping on one side of the face	1. U
_____	2. Pain intensified with deep breathing	2. U
_____	3. Disorientation	3. U
_____	4. Black stools	4. U
_____	5. Anger and denial	5. E
_____	6. Temperature above 103° F.	6. U
_____	7. Friction rub with heartbeat	7. U
_____	8. Temperature 100.8° F. on days 2 and 3	8. E
_____	9. Sudden dyspnea at night	9. U
_____	10. Occasional angina of short duration	10. E
_____	11. Anorexia	11. E
_____	12. Abdominal distention and tenderness	12. U
_____	13. Temperature 100.8° F. on days 6 and 7	13. U
_____	14. Transient paralysis on the right side	14. U
_____	15. Elevated white blood cell count	15. E
_____	16. Nausea	16. E
_____	17. Decreased arterial PO_2	17. U
_____	18. Convulsions	18. U
_____	19. Fear, depression exhibited by patient	19. E
_____	20. Elevated sedimentation rate	20. E
_____	21. Acute pain not relieved by 15-mg morphine	21. U
_____	22. Panic and hysteria exhibited by patient	22. U
_____	23. Numbers 2 and 7 are symptoms of _____.	23. pericarditis
_____	24. When this occurs after a heart attack, it usually disappears spontaneously. (True/False)	24. True

AFTER THE ACUTE PHASE (*ICC, 4th ed., pp. 20-21*)

Exercise 11

Perhaps you're studying to work in a unit called "step-down," "aftercare," or "intermediate coronary care" (ICCU)—doesn't sound very important, does it? If you've ever seen the expression of patients leaving the safe (and sometimes terrifying) cocoon of CCU—you know that ICCU is vitally important.

1. It's important to start a _____ _____ of activity and rehabilitation in ICCU.

   planned program

2. Some of the positive effects of early ambulation are: _____
   _____
   _____
   _____

   conditions cardiovascular system, prevents muscle wasting, decreases anxiety and depression

3. ICCU nurses (do/do not) have to worry about arrhythmias developing.

   do

CONVALESCENCE (*ICC, 4th ed., pp. 21-23*)

Exercise 12

Mr. Kardiac is going home tomorrow. He's excited, scared, full of questions, and he expects *you* to be full of answers. Let's listen to him. Decide how you'd answer each of his comments. Then check the suggestions in the answer column.

1. Mr. Kardiak: "Doc says I might go back to work in 2 to 3 months. Do you really think so?"
   Your answer:

   Patients who don't have any complications can usually go back to work in 2 to 3 months.

2. Mr. Kardiak: "I dunno. Old Uncle Joe never did go back to work."
   Your answer:

   Your recovery time depends on your age, general health, and heart condition.

3. Mr. Kardiak: "Doc says I gotta start walking. Me? I've never been a walker."
   Your answer:

   Walking helps so many ways. It increases your circulation and strengthens your heart. And it will help you to feel less tired and fatigued.

4. Mr. Kardiak: "I've been in this hospital 4 weeks now. How long does it take for my heart to heal?"
   Your answer:

   Generally, heart muscle heals in 6 to 8 weeks.

Listen to Mr. and Mrs. Kardiak carefully. If you suspect their apprehension is the anxiety that will make them "cardiac cripples," consult with their doctor *before* they go home.

Exercise 13

Let's take a more "clinical" look at Mr. and Mrs. Kardiak's prognosis. Review Figure 2.5 in *ICC*, 4th ed., and then fill in the blanks below. Don't worry about exact percentages. The idea is to understand the progression of LVF from class I to class IV.

1. Class I   Class II   Class III   Class IV

   (____ LVF) (_____ LVF) (_____ LVF) (_____ _____)

   no, mild, severe, cardiogenic shock

   _____% (Class I) hospital mortality rises to _____% (Class IV).

   7, 85

2. Overall hospital mortality (with CCUs) is _____ to _____%.

   15, 18

3. Another _____ to _____% of MI patients die within 12 months.

   10, 15

4. After 5 years, about _____% of MI patients will have died.

   50

3

The System of Intensive Coronary Care

THE PROBLEM OF CORONARY HEART DISEASE (*ICC, 4th ed., p. 25*)

Intensive Coronary Care, 4th ed., points out that, in the United States, almost twice as many people die from coronary heart disease as die from all forms of cancer. Think about this incredible statistic—2000 people a day die from coronary heart disease—and, no, they aren't all in their 80s or 90s. Far too many of the deaths involve hearts too young or too good to die.

Estimates indicate that there will be one million new cases of coronary heart disease annually in the United States. We, our families, friends, and neighbors, might join next year's million unless we practice some primary prevention.

Exercise 1

Ask yourself the following questions:

1. Do I smoke?

2. Do I restrict the amount of butter, eggs, whole milk, fatty meat, and cream that I eat?

3. Do I exercise regularly?

4. Do I keep my weight normal?

5. Do I find outlets for tension when I'm under emotional stress?

6. How many risk factors for CHD do I have? How about the other members of my family?

7. Do the doctors and nurses in my hospital set a good example for patients?

8. Do I teach my patients about risk factors?

THE SURGICAL APPROACH TO
THE PROBLEM (*ICC, 4th ed., p. 26*)

Exercise 2

Your patient, Mr. Angie Peck, has been admitted for surgery to receive a coronary artery bypass graft. Dr. Brusque, world-renowned coronary surgeon, spent 32 seconds yesterday explaining the procedure to the Pecks. He can't understand why they still have questions, but, because he's in surgery all day, he asks you to talk with them. He tells you, "I explained everything yesterday, but go ahead and answer any questions they have." Try to imagine yourself in the scene below and complete the nurse's explanation.

As you enter the visitor's waiting room, you are pounced upon.

Mrs. Pyranna: I'm the daughter. When's that Dr. Brusque going to talk to us? We've been waiting here for hours.

Nurse: You're done a lot of waiting these last few days, haven't you? You must be worn out. Let's all sit down and I'll see if I can help.

Mr. Pyranna: Dr. Brusque, is he . . .?

Nurse: Dr. Brusque is sorry he couldn't see you this morning. He's in surgery. He has another patient who needed the same type of surgery that Mr. Peck is scheduled for. Dr. Brusque asked me to answer questions you may have about the coronary artery bypass grafts. Do you have anything you'd like to ask me about?

Mrs. Peck: (sniffling) It seems so frightening—dangerous—cutting into the heart and . . . and all for *what?* It's not going to cure him, is it?

Nurse: There still is _____ _____ for coronary heart disease. Of the people who have this surgery_____% feel much better afterward. By this I mean, _____

_____

_____

> no cure
> 85
> they can live a more normal life without having the heart pain they had before surgery.

Mrs. Pyranna: Percents don't mean anything to Ma.

Nurse: Mrs. Peck, let me explain the 85% this way. _____

_____

_____

_____

> If 10 people had this type of surgery, 8, perhaps 9, of those people would feel much better after surgery.

Mr. Pyranna: If Dad has this surgery, will it increase his chances for living longer?

Nurse: I wish I could give you a definite answer on that. _____

_____

_____

> We need more research and experience before we have definite answers.

Mrs. Pyranna: How do they do this surgery? Dr. Brusque said they take a vein from the leg and sew it into the heart. That's not going to work. They'd have to pull an awful lot of vein up to reach clear to his heart.

Nurse: Maybe I can draw a picture that would help. But first let me explain about the leg vein. _____

_____

_____

_____

_____

_____

> The surgeon cuts a small piece of vein out of the leg and sews it into the artery in the heart that is blocked. It's like a detour—the blood can flow through the new piece of vein and avoid the the blockage.

Mrs. Peck: Oh dear, he'll be in a wheelchair the rest of his life. The would just kill him.

Nurse: Oh, no, Mrs. Peck. There are plenty of other veins to supply his leg. Look at your own leg and you'll see lots of veins.

While Mrs. Peck examines her legs you fish a note pad out of your pocket and draw a picture. Draw it and write your explanation before reading my version of this scene. Don't expect your answers to be identical to mine: They should be in your own words.

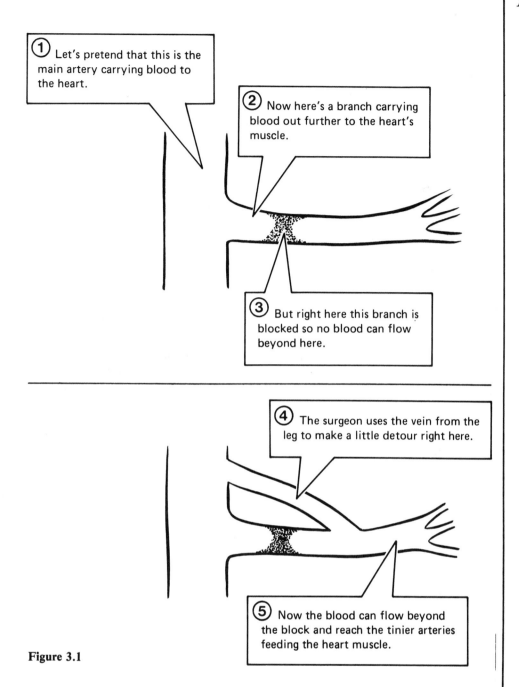

Figure 3.1

Exercise 3

Ready to try a few more questions about coronary artery bypass graft? (To save space, we'll call it CABG.)

1. In CABG a portion of the patient's _____ vein is used for the graft.

   saphenous

2. The atherosclerotic process usually involves (one/two or more) coronary arteries and that determines the number of grafts.

   two or more

3. CABG is most effective when: (a) atherosclerosis is diffuse, (b) narrowing of the artery is near the point of origin. (Choose one.)

   b

4. Label the conditions on the next page "Yes" if CABG has been demonstrated as effective treatment. Label them "No" if CABG has *not* been demonstrated as effective treatment.

a. _____ averting impending MI

b. _____ relieving angina pectoris

c. _____ increasing exercise tolerance

d. _____ stopping progression of CHD

e. _____ preventing heart failure

f. _____ prolonging life

g. _____ improving quality of life

a. no

b. yes

c. yes

d. no

e. no

f. no

g. yes

PREVENTION OF CLOTS (ICC, 4th ed., pp. 26-27)

Exercise 4

1. Clots form in arteries when the _____ become unusually _____.

platelets
sticky or adhesive

2. "Clumping" of the platelets forms the _____ for a clot.

framework

3. One theory holds that this process also may be involved in the formation of atherosclerotic _____.

plaques

4. Three drugs that inhibit platelet clumping or aggregation are: _____, _____, _____.

aspirin
Perisantine, Anturane

5. _____ seems to protect against arrhythmic deaths for _____ months after an MI (in the trials).

Anturane, 7

BETA-BLOCKING AND CALCIUM-BLOCKING DRUGS (ICC, 4th ed., pp. 27-28)

Exercise 5

1. Beta-blockers block the _____ nervous system's effects on the heart.

sympathetic

2. Thus beta-blockers would (increase/decrease) heart rate, (increase/decrease) blood pressure, (increase/decrease) the heart's work and (increase/decrease) the heart's oxygen demand.

decrease, decrease
decrease, decrease

3. Beta-blockers prevent the progression of atherosclerosis after an MI. (True/False)

False

4. Beta-blockers prolong life after recovery from an MI. (True/False)

True

5. Contradictions to the usage of beta-blockers are _____ _____ and _____ _____ _____.

heart failure
obstructive lung disease

6. Calcium-blocking drugs (increase/decrease) coronary blood flow and (increase/decrease) myocardial oxygenation.

increase, increase

7. Calcium ions enter the smooth muscle cells in order for _____ to occur.

contraction

8. Calcium-blockers _____ the entry of calcium into the cells.

block or prevent

9. Inhibiting smooth muscle contraction allows the arteries to _____.

dilate

10. This should _____ myocardial blood flow.

increase

11. Variant angina (can/cannot) be treated effectively with calcium-blockers.

can

12. Calcium-blockers also are reported effective in treating arrhythmias and heart failure. (True/False)

True

Exercise 6

PTCA— sounds like the Parent-Teachers of California, doesn't it? If ever we needed initials we need them now: percutaneous transluminal coronary angioplasty = PTCA, thank you. Using the diagram in *ICC*, 4th ed., p. 29, let's go through the PTCA process in words you might use to explain it to one of your patients.

1. The doctor inserts a _____ catheter into an artery in your arm or groin, (technically, the _____ or _____).

   guiding
   brachial, femoral

2. After the catheter is positioned in the heart, a_____ is injected to show the exact location of the blockage.

   dye

3. A _____ catheter is then inserted inside of the guide catheter.

   smaller

4. This catheter has a guide _____ and a _____ _____.

   wire, deflated balloon

5. The balloon is inflated for _____ to _____ seconds to dilate the obstructed artery.

   3, 5

6. After PTCA, the blood flow through the artery should _____ and you should feel better.

   improve or increase

THE CONCEPT AND SYSTEM OF CORONARY CARE (*ICC, 4th ed., pp. 28-32*)

Intensive Coronary Care, 4th ed., provides a clear picture of why coronary care units are necessary. Let's go over the main points in the following exercise.

Exercise 7

1. In the years BCCU (before coronary care units) at least_____ % of all patients with acute myocardial infarction died during their hospitalization.

   30

2. With coronary care units, the death rate has been reduced to about_____%.

   15

3. Previously, the most common cause of death, after a myocardial infarction, was _____.

   arrhythmia

4. The next most common cause was _____ _____.

   pump failure

5. Arrhythmias indicate an _____ disturbance of the heart.

   electrical

6. Pump failure is the result of the heart's inability to _____ _____ efficiently.

   circulate blood

7. The main cause of sudden death is _____ _____.

   ventricular fibrillation

8. This lethal arrhythmia can be terminated by _____.

   defibrillation

9. This must be accomplished within _____ minutes if life is to be saved.

   2

10. The purpose of continuous cardiac monitoring is to_____ arrhythmias.

    prevent

11. A second type of lethal arrhythmia is known as _____ _____.

    ventricular standstill

12. It can be treated by means of _____.

    pacing

13. To be effective, pacing must be started within _____.

    seconds

ARRHYTHMIAS AND PUMP FAILURE
(*ICC, 4th ed., pp. 32-33*)

Exercise 8

1. The first CCUs concentrated on _____.

   resuscitation

2. Later it was discovered that death-producing arrhythmias were usually preceded by _____ _____.

   warning arrhythmias

3. These lesser arrhythmias could often be controlled by _____ or _____.
    drugs
    pacing

4. The purpose of the CCU then became _____ of lethal arrhythmias.
    prevention

5. Presently, the CCU follows a program of _____ treatment of warning arrhythmias.
    aggressive

6. This has helped to reduce the death rate from MIs by about (1/3) (1/2) (4/5).
    (1/3)

7. CCUs have not been as successful in reducing the death rate from _____ _____.
    pump
    failure

(For the sake of space, let's refer to both left ventricular failure and cardiogenic shock by the general term *pump failure*.)

8. The successful treatment of warning arrhythmias and the unsuccessful treatment of pump failure contribute to the statistics: about _____ % of the deaths following an MI are from pump failure.
    90

9. Current treatment of pump failure includes:

A. early _____ and _____ of impending failure.
    detection, treatment

B. _____ therapy to improve pumping efficiency.
    drug

C. mechanical devices such as: _____-_____ _____ and _____ _____.
    intra-aortic balloon
    external counterpulsation

D. _____ surgery.
    bypass

REDUCTION OF MI SIZE (*ICC, 4th ed., p. 34*)

Exercise 9

1. Immediately after an MI, the two zones of myocardial damage are an inner area of severe _____ that becomes necrotic;
    ischemia

2. and an outer area of (lesser/greater) ischemia.
    lesser

3. The _____ area may recover if ischemia is controlled within _____ hours.
    outer, 3

4. The technique of using drugs to treat the border zone is called _____ _____.
    intracoronary
    thrombolysis

5. A clot is called a _____.
    thrombus

6. The purpose of this drug treatment is to _____ the size of the infarct.
    limit or reduce

7. Recovery after an MI may depend upon the _____ of the infarct and the degree of (left/right) ventricular impairment.
    size
    left

Exercise 10

In later chapters you'll learn a lot of new drug names. Let's get a head start by matching a few drugs and classifications. Write the appropriate classification (A, B, or C) in front of the drugs.

Classification	Drugs	
A—Thrombolytic	1. _____ thrombolysin	1. A
B—Beta-blocker	2. _____ metoprolol	2. B
C—Calcium-blocker	3. _____ nifedipine	3. C
	4. _____ streptokinase	4. A
	5. _____ propranolol	5. B

The triple IV that's being tested contains a _____-_____-_____ infusion.
    glucose-potassium-insulin

PRE-HOSPITAL CORONARY CARE
(ICC, 4th ed., p. 34)

Exercise 11

1. A little over (¼) (½) (¾) of MI deaths occur before hospital admission.

    ½

2. The system devised to reduce the pre-hospital mortality involved a specially equipped _____ and specially _____ _____.

    ambulance, trained personnel (i.e., EMTs)

3. When the coronary care ambulance brings the patient to the hospital, _____ _____ _____ is the next step in reducing mortality rates.

    direct admission to CCU

4. What is the procedure in your area for pre-hospital and admission?

    Check it out!

BASIC PRACTICE AND CONCEPT OF CCU
(ICC, 4th ed., pp. 35-36)

Exercise 12

1. Admission to CCU (should/should not) be determined on the basis of severity of symptoms.

    should not

2. Admission to CCU (should/should not) be determined on the basis of the level of patient care needed.

    should not

3. Admission to CCU (should/should not) be determined on the basis of history suggestive of an MI.

    should

4. Every patient suspected of having an MI (should/should not) be admitted to CCU.

    should

5. Patients usually stay in CCU _____ days, because (35%) (65%) (85%) of deaths occur within those first few days.

    5, 65%

6. Some hospitals transfer MI patients from CCU to an _____ or _____ unit rather than to the medical unit in an attempt to reduce mortality rates after the acute phase.

    intermediate subacute

7. Patients with (transmural/nontransmural) infarctions usually need to remain in CCU longer.

    transmural

8. The cornerstone of intensive coronary care is _____ _____ _____.

    prevention of complication

9. Keep in mind, many drugs used to prevent or treat complications are dangerous, so watch for overtreatment and _____ _____.

    side effects

Exercise 13

There is a diagram on page 31 of *ICC*, 4th ed., that illustrates the system of ICC. Suppose we try some role playing to get the feel of the elements involved. This play is a gross exaggeration—a parody of CCU. Please, the next time you admit a patient—prove how silly this is.

    Title: NIGHTMARE
  The Plot: To demonstrate what CCU nursing is *not* all about!
    Cast of Characters: Mr. A, a patient, the central figure
                 Mrs. Harried, Head Nurse
                 Miss Sulky, Staff Nurse
                 Mrs. A, The patient's wife
  The Scene: Night shift in a CCU

Scene1: Mr. A is raced down the hall on the ambulance cart, crashed through the doorway of CCU, and dumped into the sterile, white bed. The perspiring, panting ambulance attendants yank their sheet out from under Mr. A and then claim a ringside seat for the ensuing drama. They are finally kicked out by the CCU nurses who then, with great flair and very little finesse, proceed to strip Mr. A.

Head nurse: Hurry up—we gotta get that monitor on. Where'd the electrodes go?

Staff nurse: I though I was supposed to take the BP. You want me to go look for things or do that?

Mr. A: Am I all right?

Head nurse: Oh, crumb! This electrode won't fit into the cable.

Staff nurse: They must be trying another brand. Half the junk they get never works.

Head nurse: Where'd you put the box of broken electrical stuff? Maybe there's one in there that'll work.

Staff nurse: His BP's not so great. Want me to start an IV?

Head nurse: Are you sure you can hit the vein this time?

Mr. A: Hit who?

Staff nurse: (pouting) Well, if you don't like the way I do it, then do it yourself.

Head nurse: Oh, don't get mad. Go ahead and start the IV—you need the practice.

Mr. A: On me, she's going to practice . . . with *that* needle?

Head nurse: Hmm, this isn't *exactly* where the electrodes belong, but he's got so much hair I can't do much about it. Let's see what the pattern looks like.

Staff nurse: EECK! That's weird. I've never seen anything that looks that bad.

Mr. A: I feel sick.

Head nurse: Oh brother. I see what's wrong. I reversed the leads—his heart looks upside down! There, that's better.

Staff nurse: Boy, you sure had me worried.

Mr. A: I'm sick.

Head nurse: Look at those premature beats, one after another. Why haven't you got that IV going? If we don't treat those PVCs . . . (rolls her eyes heavenward).

Staff nurse: Well, I didn't think . . .

Head nurse: There's no time to think! How are you going to learn if you don't practice on the patients? Oh, get the bottle ready—I'll start it myself!

Mr. A: Start what?

Head nurse: Have you called x-ray? Lab? ECG? And what about the doctor?

Staff nurse: (goes to the phone muttering) Thinks I'm an octopus.

Head nurse: (softly) More like a dumb bunny.

Mr. A: Isn't my doctor here?

Head nurse: (stopping to look at him for the first time) In the middle of the night? Are you kidding?

There's a knock at the door.

Head nurse: See who's there, will you? I haven't found any veins at all.

Mr. A: Why don't I have any veins? Am I *that* sick?

Staff nurse: (grumbling) I'm supposed to be a secretary, maid, doorman .. (she opens the door)

Mrs. A and children push in.

Mrs. A: How is he? Can I see him? Will he live?

Staff nurse: (regally) Mrs. A, this is an Intensive Coronary Care Unit. Visiting hours are posted on the door. Our first responsibility here is to save the patient's life. Now, how can I do that if I'm standing here talking with you?

Mrs. A: (humbled and frightened) Oh dear, I'm sorry—so sorry. But please, can you tell me—is he okay? Will he live?

Staff nurse: (stiffly) I'm not allowed to give out any information. You'll have to ask his doctor. We'll allow you to see him for 2 minutes when we finish the admission procedures. Incidentally, have you given the Admissions Office your health insurance policy number? (Hustles Mrs. A out, then slams the door.)

Mr. A: (who has been watching his bedside monitor, jumps when the IV needle strikes home) Look at that—that little light jumped all over! Am I okay?

Staff nurse: (returning to bedside). You've gotta lie still, you know. You can't jump all over or it'll do that every time you move.

(Mr. A says nothing but lies absolutely rigid from then on.)

Head nurse: Did you get the doctor?

Staff nurse: Yeah.

Head nurse: Well, what'd you tell him?

Staff nurse: That he had a new patient. He was so sleepy. He told me to put it in the stall and feed it some grain. (giggles)

Head nurse: Honestly! Did you give him the vitals and tell him we've got PVCs?

Staff nurse: He didn't ask. But he did ask if it was bad enough for him to come right over.

Head nurse: What'd you tell him?

Staff nurse: That I wasn't a doctor so I really couldn't answer that.

Head nurse: That's a good one. What'd he say?

Staff nurse: He swore.

After reading this play you should know what CCU nurses should *not* be. But what *should* they be? *ICC*, 4th ed., describes the basic responsibilities of a CCU nurse as follows.

Exercise 14

1. The nurse must be able to _____ ECG changes and appreciate their significance.

   interpret

2. Through careful _____ of the patient the nurse repeatedly assesses the clinical condition.

   observation

3. The nurse must be capable of making _____ about a course of action.

   decisions

4. The nurse helps in caring not only for the patient's physical condition but also in supporting his or her _____ or _____ health.

   emotional, psychological

4

The Coronary Care Unit and the Staff

Chapter 4 is one of the most delightful in *ICC,* 4th ed., because it talks about you, the CCU nurse. Read and enjoy it! If you're blessed with the role of staffing a CCU or providing continuing education for CCU nurses, you'll be especially pleased with the new material Dr. Meltzer and his colleagues have provided.

Perhaps you're wondering if you should become a CCU nurse. Read this chapter and see if you can imagine yourself in the role *after* you've completed a CCU training program. If you feel inadequate, remember, we all did before we completed CCU training. And many of us have enough humility (or honesty) to still feel inadequate.

UNIT AND STAFF (*ICC, 4th ed., pp. 39-54*)

Exercise 1

Chapter 4 of the Manual does not lend itself to questions and answers. After you have read it, we'll discuss a few things from our viewpoint as nurses.

A few of you may have the dubious/delightful/delirious privilege of helping set up a new CCU. Here are some scenarios.

1. Here comes the hospital administrator, Mr. Stuffer. He says, "You need a specially trained RN and an LPN for 4 cardiacs?! Haven't got them. I'll put 2 un- trained RNs in. That won't do? Okay, 2 untrained RNs and I'll find you that LPN. You'd better accept that; after all, it's more staff than any other place in the hospital has." And off he stomps. His CCU is stuffed, not staffed! (Your new CCU has special equipment; it needs specially trained nurses to run it.)

2. How do you select the nurses for this special training? Ms. Purr Swaytion, the Director of Nurses, is selecting her staff—listen: "Imogene, we'll send you to that 2-week CCU course so you can be Head Nurse. Now, now . . . after all we've done for you, this is the very least you can do for us. And, Gertrude, you'll be in charge of pm's. Imogene will teach you; we can't afford to send you both. My dear, you won't refuse, not if you remember your annual good-behavior raise." (Coercion seldom creates good CCU nurses.)

3. Dr. Meltzer and his colleagues describe the desirable qualities of a CCU nurse in some detail. If you have dozens of applicants, then use their criteria to select the best ones. Otherwise, where do you find potential CCU nurses? Have you thought of the nurse who is bored by routine? The one who likes a challenge? The one who hates making schedules and being a "desk jockey"? The one who handles any new assignment well but never volunteers?

   How do you convince these nurses that CCU may be just what they'd love? How can nurses who have never been inside a unit decide if they'd like it? Maybe you can arrange a visit to a nearby CCU; most hospitals are happy to show off their units. And CCU nurses themselves are usually good recruiters because most of them love their units. If you are wondering about being a CCU nurse yourself, visiting a unit may help you decide.

4. The Manual says that a CCU should be "autonomous" and not be turned into an overflow area for all intensive care patients. What happens when this rule is violated? CCU's phone is ringing; let's answer it and see: "Yes, a new MI to admit? I'm sorry, we're full. We have one alcoholic, two drug overdoses, a stroke, and a terminal CA. Oh, you'll admit the MI to Peds then?"

   One way to combat this is to get a nurse on the planning committee and the committee responsible for operating the CCU. The nurse realizes it's hard to monitor an MI when all hands, including the cleaning lady's, are busy holding a drug overdose patient in bed. Why shouldn't the nurse have a say in the operation of the unit? And, if you can't achieve this bit of utopia, then don't hesitate to voice your opinion—CCU beds should be available for *coronary* patients, not as a catch-all.

5. You have a say in design and equipment, but you're confused. Run, don't walk, to every CCU in your area and quiz the NURSES on what they'd change in their own set-up if they had the opportunity. Collect pros and cons on various unit floor plans: open, partitioned, hallways, etc.

   Equipment? Many manufacturers send their representatives to prospective clients, and often they'll demonstrate their products for you. Ask if they'll leave the monitor, or whatever the item is, for a week or so—to give you a chance to familiarize yourself with it. Use your imagination and test the equipment: You're at the bedside of a cardiac arrest patient. Can you start the monitor's write-out function from here? Or, if you've missed something that flew across the screen, is there a memory tape? Practice using the equipment and ask questions—nobody should have to buy "a pig in a poke." And find out how good the manufacturer's service is *after* you buy their equipment—your janitor is probably not capable of repairing the defibrillator if it starts shooting sparks.

6. All hospitals, even hospitals without CCUs, need crash carts. (*See ICC, 4th ed., pp. 43-44*, for a list of equipment and supplies found on crash carts). Many hospitals store their supplies in a cart designed for a radial saw, and often a tool box or a fishing tackle box is used as an emergency drug kit. Funny thing—they work beautifully.

   One thing you must insist on is that NO ONE borrow from the emergency supplies just because they're handy. You need a check list and people assigned to keep track of the crash cart and drug box supplies on a regular basis. It's too late to begin searching for a drug once the emergency has occurred.

7. You'll probably have very little say in training the medical staff. But, surprisingly, you'll often find yourself teaching doctors who are not specialists in coronary care. Offer your suggestions in as pleasant and inoffensive a manner as possible and you can be an effective doctor—teacher. Remember, YOU are the specialist in patient care, and even a cardiologist can learn from you!

8. In *ICC, 4th ed., pp. 50-52*, is listed the didactic material a CCU course should cover in training the CCU nurse (somehow I'd rather be educated than trained, how about you?). It's beautiful—push hard for every lecture listed!

9. If your unit is new and your nurses inexperienced, can you arrange to obtain some clinical experience (or at least observe the operations) in a neighboring CCU?

10. Ongoing education is extremely important. I'm in favor of it—1000%. But once your unit is staffed and running, do your doctors lose interest in further teaching? Then organize the nurses! There are films, books, conferences—share and study. If necessary, you can make ongoing education a do-it-yourself project. And you must continue learning; with today's knowledge explosion, standing still means falling behind.

   One last thought: after you've been in a CCU a while and your own importance threatens to overwhelm you (which happens to most of us), remember this:

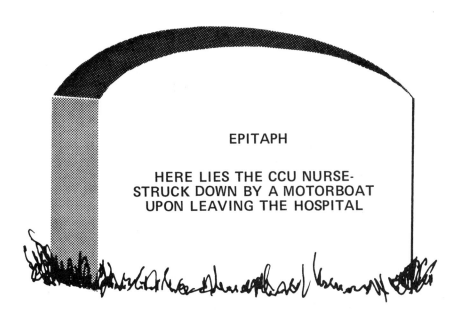

EPITAPH

HERE LIES THE CCU NURSE-
STRUCK DOWN BY A MOTORBOAT
UPON LEAVING THE HOSPITAL

Exercise 2

Take a good look at the list of drugs stocked in CCU at the Presbyterian-University of Pennsylvania Medical Center pp. 45-46. Remember the drug cards you made when you were in nursing school? Why not start making cards with these drugs? You've got a lot of drugs to become familiar with, so why wait until Chapter 16? Pick drugs from each category that your hospital stocks. Get help from your pharmacist or CCU nurses and make friends with a new drug.

TERMINOLOGY REVIEW (*ICC, 4th ed., Chapters 3-4*)

Exercise 3

Listed here is a series of definitions and fill-in-the-blank statements. First, write the answers where indicated. Then, if you want to have some fun, try to find the answers in the *Word Rounds*. The words read from left to right, top to bottom, and diagonally. You simply circle the answers, some of which are two-word combinations. One answer has been circled to show you how the game works.

Perfect Score = 20 points. Three words appear twice in the *Word Rounds*; if you find both, then score: Super Perfect = 23 points. (Answers to *Word Rounds* appear on the next page.)

P	K	O	S	C	I	L	L	O	S	C	O	P	E	C	J	G
S	R	T	R	D	I	N	T	E	R	M	E	D	I	A	T	E
U	D	I	D	A	C	T	I	C	K	Z	R	V	K	R	L	E
D	Z	M	M	O	N	I	T	O	R	L	E	Z	G	D	H	K
D	B	S	W	A	Z	D	E	L	E	G	A	T	E	I	B	M
E	G	T	A	B	R	V	L	M	N	O	V	T	R	O	R	N
N	V	A	R	R	H	Y	T	H	M	I	A	S	V	G	K	Z
D	Z	B	N	C	R	D	P	A	C	E	M	A	K	E	R	S
E	R	L	I	O	D	I	L	R	N	P	K	G	R	N	Z	D
A	Z	E	N	N	T	D	O	L	E	T	H	A	L	I	G	M
T	V	H	G	F	H	A	V	B	Q	V	K	R	N	C	H	D
H	B	T	N	E	G	C	D	K	L	L	E	D	Z	K	L	G
M	A	T	U	R	I	T	Y	V	G	E	B	N	D	Z	R	V
R	D	E	M	E	T	I	C	L	O	T	S	D	T	E	A	M
V	K	A	R	N	Z	C	K	R	V	H	G	A	W	I	R	V
P	D	M	V	C	L	I	N	I	C	A	L	B	O	M	O	A
Z	A	B	D	E	F	I	B	R	I	L	L	A	T	I	O	N

1. You have _____ minutes to defibrillate a patient after ventricular fibrillation begins.

two

2. Control of risk factors from childhood on to decrease CHD: _____ _____.

primary prevention

3. Capable of causing death: _____.

lethal

4. Part of a cardiac monitor: _____.

oscilloscope

5. _____ causes 1/3 of all deaths in the United States.

CHD

6. Electric shock used to treat ventricular fibrillation: _____.

defibrillation

7. Equipment that aids the nurse in observing the patient: _____.

monitor

8. A physician-nurse _____ cares for the patient in CCU.

team

9. Ventricular fibrillation and ventricular standstill: _____ _____.

sudden death

10. Subacute care after the critical CCU stage: _____.

intermediate

11. Type of arrhythmias that must be treated to prevent lethal arrhythmias: _____ _____.

warning arrhythmias

12. Prevention of _____ formation may be accomplished by anticoagulants.

clot

13. Abnormal heart rhythms: _____..

arrhythmias

14. Sites in the heart that initiate heartbeats: _____.

pacemakers

15. The physician must _____ responsibility to the nurse.

delegate

16. Rational, steadfast: a desirable CCU nurse quality: _____.

stable

17. Instructional elements—necessary part of CCU course: _____.

didactic

18. Desired state of emotional development: _____. maturity

19. Applied experience—a necessary part of CCU course: _____. clinical

20. Group meetings for continuing ongoing CCU education: _____. conference

Answers

P K O S C I L L O S C O P E C J G
S R T R D I N T E R M E D I A T E
U D I D A C T I C K Z R V K R L E
D Z M M O N I T O R L E Z G D H K
D B S W A Z D E L E G A T E I B M
E G T A B R V L M N O V T R O R N
N V A R R H Y T H M I A S V G K Z
D Z B N C R D P A C E M A K E R S
E R L I O D I L R N P K G R N Z D
A Z E N N T D O L E T H A L I G M
T V H G F H A V B Q V K R N C H D
H B T N E G C D K L L E D Z K L G
M A T U R I T Y V G E B N D Z R V
R D E M E T I C L O T S D T E A M
V K A R N Z C K R V H G A W I R V
P D M V C L I N I C A L B O M O A
Z A B D E F I B R I L L A T I O N

39

5

Coronary Care Nursing

NURSING SKILLS (*ICC, 4th ed., pp. 55-61*)

"I'm a Coronary Care Nurse." What will it mean when you can say that? It means hours of study and lots of hard, devoted work. It means hearing the family say, "We feel safe with you here." And after an emergency, when the patient says, "Hey, I'm still alive," it means indescribable ecstasy. Read all of Chapter 5 in *ICC*, 4th ed. It's an interesting chapter because it's about you and your role. Be aware of how much reliance is placed on the judgment of the nurse. Good judgment has replaced rigid schedules.

"You, the beginner, are unique. Use your own knowledge and skills, and let's build on those." That's a quote from the Preface of this book, in case you might have forgotten it. *You* are the best judge of your own current level of expertise. By now you should have a fairly good idea of where you're headed.

Exercise 1

The following table, the outline of nursing duties and responsibilities, is based on information in Chapter 5, *ICC*, 4th ed. Assess your current skills and knowledge, then decide where you'd like them to be. Write down your ideas on how you can develop the skills and knowledge you would like to have. You might want to refer to this chart periodically to check on your progress as a CCU nurse.

Table 5.1. Outline of Nursing Duties and Responsibilities

Areas of competency	Present level	Desired level	How to get there
Assessing Clinical Status			
ECG monitoring			
General observation			
Left ventricular failure			
Cardiogenic shock			
Hemodynamic monitoring			
CVP (Central venous pressure)			
Swan-Ganz catheter			
Anticipating & Preventing Complications			
Establish & maintain IV			
Administer oxygen			
Diagnose & treat			
warning arrhythmias			
Monitor pacemakers			
Emergency Treatment & Resuscitation			
Defibrillation			
CPR			
Assisted respiration			
Manual bag			
Respirator			
Rotating tourniquets			
Diagnostic Procedures			
Record 12-lead ECGs			
Perform venipuncture			
Assist in obtaining arterial blood gases			
General Nursing Care			
Develop & implement a nursing care plan			
Emotional Support			
Observe			
Listen			
Intervene			
Communicating			
With patient/family			
With physician			
With nurses			
Collecting & Recording Data			
Nursing history			
Interviewing patient			
Record patient history			
Admitting assessment			
Document arrhythmias			

42

Table 5.1. Outline of Nursing Duties and Responsibilities (cont'd.)

Areas of competency	Present level	Desired level	How to get there
Collecting & Recording Data (cont'd.)			
Monitor drug therapy			
Effects			
Side effects			
Record dosage			
Nursing notes			
Assess			
Record			
Teaching Skills			
Role modeling			
Teaching skills			
Patient Teaching			
Planning			
Assessing			
Implementing			

ADMITTING THE PATIENT (*ICC, 4th ed., pp. 62-65*)

Let's try admitting a patient. Dr. Hart calls and says, "I'm sending a patient over from the office. I think he might be an MI, but he's not in severe pain right now. Admit him and then call me."

Exercise 2

Answer these questions, and then read the discussion that follows.

1. The very first thing you'll do when the patient arrives is _____
_____.

ATTACH THE MONITOR. No 5-minute welcoming speech; don't demonstrate the call bell system; don't present the complimentary admission kit; don't even take his TPR—get the monitor on. Know your equipment so well that you can think about the patient's feelings and not the hardware connections.

2. While you're doing this you should _____
_____.

EXPLAIN WHAT THE EQUIPMENT IS ALL ABOUT. But don't expect him to remember; his anxiety level at this point is too high for that. During the rest of his stay in CCU, encourage him to ask questions and repeat explanations as often as necessary.

3. He may develop an arrhythmia at any time, so take an _____
_____.

ADMISSION MONITOR STRIP—stat. Later on when the doctor says, "Was he having these PVCs on admission?" you can show him exactly what the initial cardiac rhythm was.

4. What should you write on this admission monitor slip? (This isn't in *ICC*, 4th ed., so three cheers if you get it.) _____
_____.

WRITE THE PATIENT'S NAME, THE DATE, AND THE TIME ON THE STRIP. Many nurses also write the doctor's name on it.

5. While you're admitting him, what else should you be doing? _____
_____.

OBSERVE THE PATIENT AND GATHER CLINICAL INFORMATION. If you know your equipment, you can attach it automatically and spend your time talking with the patient. Determine [1] type and degree of pain, [2] location of pain, [3] symptoms of heart failure or shock, and [4] general appearance and condition.

6. He may need emergency cardiac drugs, so it's a good idea to _____
_____.

START AN IV AS SOON AS THE MONITOR IS ON. If you have a helper, then

7. When would you call the doctor? _____
_____.

do both procedures at once. Although you may be able to identify an arrhythmia and know how to treat it, you're still lost without an IV for emergency drug treatment. Get this lifeline in place in a hurry.

AFTER YOU ATTACH THE MONITOR, HAVE THE IV IN PLACE, TAKE VITAL SIGNS, AND ASSESS THE PATIENT'S CONDITION. (In other words, WHEN YOU HAVE COMPLETED numbers 1-6 above.) Then you have worthwhile information to give the doctor.

8. The doctor orders a 12-lead ECG. Why? _____
_____.

TO DIAGNOSE AN MI. The monitor only tells you about arrhythmias.

Exercise 3

You've just settled your first patient when the ambulance team calls. "We're bringing in a bad one, don't know if he'll make it." What do you do? Panic and get it over with. Then prepare for anything.

1. In preparing for the patient, you'd put at the bedside the _____
_____.

CRASH CART (including the defibrillator). Screen it if you feel it looks too frightening, but have the defibrillator plugged in and ready to go.

2. When the patient arrives, the first thing you'll do is _____
_____.

GET THE MONITOR ELECTRODES ON. If the house doctor wants to examine the patient and Respiratory Therapy wants to work with him, fine—but you shove in there and get the monitor working.

3. How about undressing the patient first? _____
_____.

NO, INDEED! I saw a 42-year-old man go into cardiac arrest while we were undressing him. I'm convinced that shoes and pants don't count. All you need is a bare chest with electrodes on, and you're set to save a life.

4. While you're putting the monitor on should you _____ to the patient what you're doing and why? Even if he's in critical condition? _____
_____.

EXPLAIN
Yes, maybe he can hear you even if he is too weak to talk.

5. Why rush to start an IV? _____
_____.

EMERGENCY DRUGS MAY BE NEEDED—undoubtedly *will* be needed. And the IV line will be instantly available.

Exercise 4

There's so much to discuss about the nursing care of the CCU patient; maybe we can do it best if you'll join me in my favorite unit. I've oriented many new nurses, and the flexibility of the nursing routines always seems to frighten them. (But then, I may be too relaxed; why don't you decide for yourself?) I'll play the role of the head nurse (HN) and you be the new nurse (NN). You can evaluate both roles as well as answer the questions. Don't be afraid to criticize.

Report is over and the 7-3 shift day is beginning.

NN: How often should I take Mr. Karkiak's BP?

HN: Let's see. The night shift took it every 4 hours; they felt he needed the sleep. Suppose we take it every 2 hours unless his condition changes.

NN: Aren't there any rules about taking BPs?

HN: Yes, but we use our own judgment, too.

QUESTION: How do you feel about the head nurse's answers?

HN: I also assigned Mrs. MI to you.

NN: Yes, I think I'll give her a bath first.

HN: I wonder if Mrs. MI really needs a bath . . .

NN: Everybody needs a daily bath.

HN: Not necessarily. Remember the night shift said Mrs. MI had a miserable night? They just got her to sleep about 5 AM. She's had so much pain, why don't we let her rest?

NN: If we wait, I won't get her bath done before 10. And suppose we have another admission?

HN: You don't have to be done with baths by 10 to be a good CCU nurse. If the patient needs to rest all day, the PM shift will sponge her off and change linen.

QUESTION: How do you feel about this advice?

NN: I'll do Mr. Kardiak's bath, then.

HN: Fine. You can give him some passive exercises during his bath, too.

NN: What? I thought he was supposed to rest. Won't exercise make his heart work harder?

HN: Yes, but he still needs to maintain the range of motion in his joints. You can help while you're washing him merely by raising his arms and moving his legs up and down and in and out a couple times. Watch his monitor while you're doing it, and, if his heart rate increases, then slow down.

NN: Okay, I'll do him first.

HN: Why don't you ask him when he'd like his bath? You know, it must be awfully hard for a big, strong man to have no choice in the matter. If you can let him "direct the traffic," it helps him feel he is still in control of his life.

QUESTION: Why not have a physical therapist do range of motion at this point? What about patient involvement in planning and choosing?

HN: By the way, did you notice anything about Mrs. MI's intake and output at report?

NN: Well, she's on an 8-hour "I and O."

HN: Anything else?

NN: It seems to me her output was rather low.

HN: Yes. Do you think we should watch her "I and O" more carefully?

NN: Okay, I'll keep an eye on her Foley.

HN: Why don't we connect a urometer to her Foley and do hourly urines?

NN: Hourly? Do we have an order for that?

HN: No, not a specific order, but let's keep an hourly record of intake and output anyway. As soon as we're sure her output is decreasing, we'll notify the doctor.

NN: He'll probably order a diuretic.

HN: Possibly. If he does, I'd like you to empty the urometer and start measuring all over again after you give her the diuretic.

NN: Why?

HN: It helps to know just what her output is a half an hour, an hour, and so forth after a diuretic is first given.

NN: I see; then the doctor can evaluate how effective it is.

QUESTION: Are we anticipating too much? Going beyond the nurse's role?

At 7, 9, and 11 AM, Mr. Kardiak's blood pressure was satisfactory; he seemed fine during his bath. Lunch came at 11:30 AM.

HN: Would you feed Mr. Kardiak?

NN: He wants to feed himself.

HN: Oh, did you explain that sometimes the heart works extra hard during meals and we just want to help it rest?

NN: Well, not really.

HN: You might also mention that you enjoy having a chance to talk with him while you're feeding him.

NN: Um-mm.

HN: However, use your own judgment. Some men are so upset by being fed—makes them feel like babies—that the agitation isn't worth it.

QUESTION: Could you improve on the head nurse's answers?

NN: There's something funny about Mr. Kardiak.

HN: Exactly what do you mean?

NN: Well, he seemed vague, preoccupied. I can't put my finger on it, but he's just different.

HN: That may be important. Have you checked his BP?

NN: It isn't due until 1 PM.

HN: Would you take it now, please? You've discovered that something's wrong, and we need all the clues we can get to determine what it is.

QUESTION: Can you see the importance of being a thinking nurse?

EMOTIONAL SUPPORT OF THE MI PATIENT *(ICC, 4th ed., pp. 68-72)*

ICC, 4th ed., has excellent information on emotional responses and emotional support. Read it carefully. As nurses, we see these reactions in every one of our patients, and we should know them well. The following poem will help us to take a closer look.

FACES OF FEAR

How do we know the faces of fear that we see in our own CCU?
The mouths, do they open and close on the words
I'm afraid!
Will you help me?
I'm scared!
Not very often . . .
Not me, not to me
Strong, robust, roving, roaming.
To have to be fed,
Tethered down in this bed.
I'm a puppet with strings to my heart.
Ashen wife, tears held back.
They lie, those tests,
It's someone else.
Really, just somethin' I et.

47

Why me, why to me?
I'm a father with children,
Wife, life, love, longing . . . leaving?
Yes me, yes to me but . . .
Perhaps to stop smoking,
Be kind, gentle, loving?
Give my eyes or my kidneys . . .
Are they taking livers these days?
How 'bout it, God . . .
Two more years?
It's a deal?
What do we do with these faces of fear that we meet in our own CCU?
Our mouths, do they open and close on the words
You're afraid.
Can I help you?
I care.
Well, they should . . .
Fear all alone is so AWFUL—
Together, perhaps, not as bad?
—*Mary Bayer*

Together now, let's consider the emotional reactions we see in our patients.

FACES OF ANXIETY

Mr. Mild Anxiety: He's one of the rarest patients we see in a CCU. He has reached the stage where he has accepted his condition and has begun to adjust to it.

Mr. Moderate Anxiety: He stares out the window and is quiet and withdrawn during morning care. At bathtime he complains about the noisy night shift, fusses about the hospital breakfast, and argues that he should be able to sit in the chair and watch TV. Later he apologizes for being a bother, but soon he is complaining of a backache and a headache. "And, by the way, when is that doctor coming back—next year?"

Mrs. Severe Anxiety: She scrutinizes your face as you check her vital signs. "What's my blood pressure now? *Exactly.* Isn't that higher than last time? One point? Two points? Say, is this thing in my arm working? I don't see it dripping. Are you sure? It was going faster yesterday." She examines each pill you give her, turns it over, feels the groove, smells it: "Are you sure this is *my* pill?" She pulls and picks at the covers, "I just can't rest. This bed—I can't stand it much longer. Can't you *do* something, Nurse?"

Mr. Panic: He's scared to death. He jumps each time you approach. His quivering and fidgeting repeatedly set off the monitor alarms. One day he leaps out of bed and, with the IV site dripping blood and the monitor cables flapping behind him, runs frantically down the hall.

Mr. Denial: "Heart attack? That's crazy. That's crazy. Why, back in '58, I had something just like this—one of them hernias. You know, where your stomach crawls up into your chest? I'll be okay, soon's I get home and take some baking soda. Stay in bed for a stomach ache? That's stupid. There's nothing wrong with me."

Mr. Angry: "I've never seen such a bunch of lousy nurses. Why that big fat night nurse, she's so mean! 'No sleeping pills after 5 AM,' she says. Then she jabs me with the dullest needle she can find. And those giggly evening nurses—they just care about their dates and hairdos. That Head Nurse is so high and mighty, she just cares about the equipment—wouldn't notice if I was dead. You better believe I'm never coming back to this dump again! I'll die first."

Mr. Bargainer: "God won't let me die yet. I've got kids to raise. Surely He'll let me finish that. I'll start going to church regularly and give my tithe. Say, Nurse, you sure look nice today. The wife's gonna bring in some candy—you be sure to come by when she's here. You'll be here when I need you, won't you?" He bargains with you or the doctors, but most of all with God.

These are some of the faces of fear that you'll see with all their subtle shadings and variations. What do we do about them? Here's a plan that we can put to use in our nursing practice.

1. Watch for the faces of fear. Be alert to the actions and reactions of your individual patients. OBSERVE!

2. Listen to your patients actively, positively.

3. Act as the patients' advocate in helping them deal with their environment, the other members of the health team, their family, and themselves.

This means we're going to do three simple things in helping our patients: observe, listen, and act. To begin, concentrate on *watching*. Everyone you meet, all of your patients—be alert to what they look like, how they express themselves, and how they handle their feelings. Under your nurse's cap (or in place of one), develop antennae that receive patient signals.

Perhaps you've already seen many of the faces of fear. You may have seen the patient who *1)* thinks his heart will stop if the monitor stops, *2)* thinks interference on the monitor is a sign of heart damage, *3)* thinks the monitor's On light is a danger signal, *4)* is sure that IVs are used only on dying patients, *5)* is sure that frequent checks of vital signs mean he's critical, *6)* is afraid to have any but the "best" nurses touch him, *7)* is afraid to move or turn.

Exercise 5

You've probably seen other reactions you could add to this list. If so, it's time to proceed to the next skill: *listening*. All of us realize the importance of communicating: we talk *and* listen to our patients. But perhaps we can improve the way we communicate.

Mark with a plus (+) the phrases that you would use in talking with patients. Mark with a zero (0) those you feel shouldn't be used.

_____ 1. "You look rather upset."

_____ 2. "I know how frightening a hospital can be."

_____ 3. "It must be hard to face being inactive."

_____ 4. "Of course you'll get well."

_____ 5. "Many of our patients feel like you do. I understand how you feel."

_____ 6. "It must be difficult to be cooped up in bed."

_____ 7. "Come now, let's think about cheerful things."

_____ 8. "It must be tough to feel that way."

_____ 9. "You'll feel better tomorrow."

_____ 10. "You seem a little tense and jittery."

_____ 11. "You have a good doctor and well-trained nurses. Don't worry."

_____ 12. "Would you like to talk about it?"

_____ 13. "Now just relax, we'll do the worrying."

_____ 14. "We'll watch your monitor, don't you worry about it."

_____ 15. "Uh-mm, Oh . . . , Uh huh . . ."

_____ 16. "I understand . . ."

Answers and Comments

__+__ 1. Sounds blunt, doesn't it? But if the patient does seem upset, it's an honest opener. He can confirm or deny it. Often he'll say, "No, I'm not upset, but I'm sure worried about . . ."

__0__ 2. You don't know how frightening—or painful, or difficult—it is for him. And that's what he really cares about.

49

_+_ 3. "It must be hard to . . ." is a great opener if you finish with words or ideas the patient himself has expressed. If your patient says, "I hate this hospital," you can say, "It must be hard to have to be here and feel that way." Then hang on to your cap, you may hear more than you can comfortably handle. But remember, it's like ventilating a stale-smelling room; the odor will improve.

_0_ 4. Oh yeah? And how do you know? Reassure the patient, don't patronize him. These are adults, not children.

_0_ 5. First you reduce him to just another statistic—one of many—then you play God. If he asks, "Have you ever seen anybody this bad?" try saying "It must be hard to feel so bad."

_+_ 6. "It must be difficult to . . ." is another great opener. It gives the patient the opportunity to evaluate for himself and to let you know.

_0_ 7. One of the best ways to turn your patient into a clam. He'll figure you think his thoughts are bad and you don't want to hear nasty things. So he'll just shut up.

_+_ 8. "It must be tough to . . ." is as good an opener as those in numbers 3 and 6.

_0_ 9. And what if he doesn't? What does that make you?

_+_ 10. An honest reflection of how he looks to you. It tells the patient you're willing to listen to how he *does* feel.

_0_ 11. So did all the ex-presidents of the United States, and how many of them are alive today? If the patient asks, "What do you think of my doctor?" Give him a *positive,* objective answer. (You can, even if you *can't* stand his doctor!) "He's well-trained," "His patients all do well," "He comes any time you need him," "I like him," "He's my favorite," are all good responses.

_+_ 12. Excellent! "It" means whatever the patient wants it to mean—an invitation for the patient to select the topic. A good follow-up to numbers 3, 6, and 8. If the patient says, "It sure is tough," you can ask, "Would you like to talk about it?"

_0_ 13. He'd relax if he could. Prompting won't help.

_0_ 14. Same as 13. Yes, he needs to know you watch the monitor; he should know you can see it from the desk, too. But leave off the "don't worry."

_+_ 15. Noncommittal, but soothing, comforting sounds. If skillfully used, they show the patient you're listening, not planning tomorrow's dinner. They encourage him to continue without your passing judgment on what he says. Skillful use takes practice; otherwise you sound bored or uncaring.

_0_ 16. A phrase you should eliminate from your nursing vocabulary. *Nobody* on earth fully understands you, or me, or your patient.

Exercise 6

Think of the faces of fear you've seen in your patients. What one fear do they all share? Fear of the unknown, right? It's the same fear that makes us cold and sweaty in the dentist's office or at a meeting when we're asked to speak.

What can you do to reduce some of the unknowns surrounding your patient? You do many things consciously and unconsciously. List some of them before you check the list below.

Here are a few of my ideas that might be helpful. Add them to your list if you think they are useful.

UNKNOWN STAFF

Introduce yourself to the patient. If you have a name, you're a "person," not just some nurse.

Eliminate unnecessary rotation of assignments among nurses.

Introduce new staff members to the patient.

UNKNOWN ENVIRONMENT

Explain to each patient the things he sees about him. Does he know that the red light on the monitor means that it is "on," not that he's in danger?

Does he think that IVs are only used on the dying?

If the defibrillator must be at his bedside, can you curtain it? Many a night nurse remembers a patient with bulging eyeballs staring at that "electric chair" machine.

LACK OF ORIENTATION TO TIME AND PLACE

Do you provide a clock and calendar in the unit? No wonder he's confused as to what day or time it is.

Reorient him frequently: "It's 10 AM, and I have a pill for you." "It's 3 PM and I need to see how much is left in your IV bottle."

Does he wear glasses or a hearing aid? What an out-of-focus, frightening world it must be without them.

UNREASSURING REASSURANCES

"You're doing just fine." So why is he still in CCU? Try being specific: "Your pulse is more regular today." "You don't seem short of breath after your bath this morning." "You sat up 5 minutes longer today." Give him tangibles so that he can measure and say to himself, "Yes, I am doing better." The family needs these measuring sticks, too, because they also wonder if he's really improving.

Now we'll look at the specific faces of fear to see how we can provide better nursing care for them:

Anxiety can be decreased through activity: Why do you pace the floor or pleat a gum wrapper when you're tense? Since physical activity is denied these patients, they can at least be allowed a voice in the activities of planning, directing, and choosing what to do when they feel up to it. This gives patients a sense of worth. When we deny them any say in their daily activities, aren't we suggesting that they are mentally as well as physically deficient?

Panic or near-panic often shows itself in abnormally exaggerated ways. Some patients may need the protection of drugs and restraints, but often a "sitter" at the bedside is enough.

Try to see the environment from the patient's point of view. That relaxing seascape may seem a swirling, threatening hurricane to him. The defibrillator or the crash cart may be "a big, black monster." Is his IV threatening to fall and crush him? Does he fly to pieces when you slam the bedpan into the bedside table or kick the footstool under the bed? If his perceptions are distorted, it may be helpful to reduce the number of stimuli he can respond to.

Denial: Don't contradict him; he only has to deny even harder. Allow him his right to deny, but in small, positive ways emphasize the reality of the situation. You might say things such as: "Your IV must stay in. The monitor still shows us that you may need some medication to help your heart," or "You look tired; may I turn this light off so you can rest?"

Bargaining: Does the patient flatter or compliment you? Maybe he's bargaining with you! Accept this stage and don't rely on his compliments to boost your ego. Then let him move out of the bargaining phase when he is ready. If he's made a bargain with God, the prayer book or rosary that you stuffed in the bottom drawer may be vitally important.

His clergyman may be able to give more support than you or the family can offer.

Anger: This is a hard one because anger is often vented on you, the nurse. It helps to remember he's not angry with you; he's mad at what's happened to him.

Possibly some of his anger is justified. After all, hospital staffs aren't perfect. However, it's more likely that the people he rages at are innocent. Battles between staff members and wars between shifts are sometimes started by the patient who is in the anger phase of adjustment. Watch it. If you wage war with this patient's ammunition, you may be shooting a paper cannon.

If the patient is venting his anger on you, understand and try to help others realize that he's angry at fate, or himself, or God—you're just handier.

Your patients will probably wear many masks of fear, changing them frequently. You won't feel lost or helpless if you practice the two phrases: "It must be hard to . . ." and "Would you like to talk about it?"

Mary Bayer, who wrote the poem "Faces of Fear," brings up one other point. "You may be confused by patients who are speaking a 'symbolic' language. You must decode their messages and return your message in their code." She tells about a patient lying absolutely rigid, arms beside her, palms up, her eyes rolling back and forth from the wall at her feet, to the wall at her right side and head, to the curtain at her left side. The patient said, "There's a wall at my feet and my head and on both sides of me." Mary replied, "It's too soon for that, isn't it?" The patient began to cry, and said, "I feel like I'm already in my casket." By using the patient's symbolic language, Mary helped her voice her fears.

Last, don't try to force your patient from one phase to the next. He moves at his own speed, and you must move with him. If you don't stifle the mechanisms or hopes of each phase, you'll provide your patient with real psychological support.

6

Cardiac Monitoring

PRINCIPLES OF CARDIAC MONITORING
(ICC, 4th ed., pp. 73-79)

Suppose you had never done any sewing. Would you buy a pattern, read through the instructions, and, without any practice, begin making a wedding dress for a friend? Idiotic, of course. But how many nurses read about monitoring and then are either too shy, embarrassed, or busy to actually practice with a monitor?

Right now you're probably saying, "But I don't know anything about monitors. I'm scared to death of them." (At least that's what I said the first time I cared for a monitored patient. Now I love it.) There are two maxims I'd like to pass on to you. The first is original; the second came from a Basic Nursing instructor before the advent of monitoring. First, the monitor is your slave; you are its master. And second, you need only to be more intelligent or more stubborn than your equipment. There will be times when you will need mastery, intelligence, and tenacity.

Intensive Coronary Care, 4th ed., stresses continuous monitoring in a special unit; but perhaps your hospital is small and patients are monitored in their rooms without a central station or special nurses. If this is the case, why not put your cardiac patients near the nurses' station? See if the cable from the patient to the monitor is long enough to set the monitor in the hallway. Everybody who walks by should look at it every time he or she passes it. If the cord is too short, ask your salesperson for a longer one. Use the beeper if it doesn't bother the patient; tune yourself in to it, and subconsciously you'll notice any changes. One point: never forget that coronary care means much, much more than cardiac monitoring, which is just one part of a nurse's responsibilities.

We'll start your introduction to cardiac monitoring in this way:

1. List the parts of a monitor as described in *ICC,* 4th ed., and then find each of these elements on the monitors used in your hospital.

2. Read the instruction manual that comes with your monitor.

3. You'll learn the most by doing, so don't just read this and nod your head; go shake hands with a monitor.

Now let's put it all together with a Monitor Game, that takes you step by step through the procedure for applying a monitor. Practice on yourself, a cohort, a patient, or even a pillow if you have to. You lose 5 points if your first monitored patient asks, "Is this the first time you've done this?"

Exercise 1

1. Find a monitor. (In some hospitals this should be worth more than one point.)   (1)

2. Got the instruction manual? Then read it.   (1)

3. Plug the power cord into the monitor. (Look again. It plugs in somewhere.)   (1)

4. You need a patient cable to run from the monitor to your patient. Attach it to the monitor. (Check the instruction manual.)   (5)

5. Where are the patient leads that connect the cable to the patient's electrodes? (They may or may not already be attached to the electrodes.) You should find 3 skinny wires that plug into a connector on the free end of the cable. (5 points when you can plug them in without fumbling.)   (5)

6. Now look at your electrodes. They're usually prepackaged. You say Central Supply will kill you if you open too many for practice? Then try to get some accidentally opened ones or one set just for practice. Read the instructions. You must attach the lead wires to the skin electrodes. Do you need conductive jelly, paste, or are the electrodes "pre-gooped"?   (5)

7. Where do the electrodes go on the patient? Let's do a conventional lead. Say to yourself: "Cross your heart. One high on the right, one low on the left." (*ICC*, 4th ed., has pictures of the electrode positions on page 77.) The ground electrode goes anywhere that's convenient. (On the patient, that is, not the bed!)   (5)

    A. Shave the patient, if necessary. Clean the area with alcohol.   (5)

    B. Connect electrodes to wires.   (5)

    C. Put "goop" on the electrodes, if needed.   (5)

    D. Attach electrodes to the patient.   (5)

(*Note:* You can do D before B, but some patients complain that it hurts when you snap (push hard) the electrode wires onto the electrode pads on their chest. Try it on yourself both ways.)

8. Now step back and admire your work. What? No monitor picture?

    A. Did you give the machine time to warm up?   (1)

    B. Is the plug in the wall socket?   (1)

    C. Is the cable plugged into the monitor?   (1)

    D. Is the patient cable in place?   (1)

    E. Are the wires on the cable firmly inserted into the connector?   (1)

    F. Are the electrodes on the wires?   (1)

    G. Are the electrodes on the patient?   (1)

    H. All right—did you turn the monitor on?   (1)

9. Is there a Sensitivity or Gain dial on your machine? Try it. See what it does.   (1)

10. How about a Position Selector switch? Try it, too. (Don't worry if your monitor doesn't have one.)   (1)

11. Too much electrical interference? (The ECG pattern looks like a satin stitch on the sewing machine—60 little lines per second.) You have to get rid of any interference.

    A. Sometimes just changing to a different wall outlet will help.   (1)

    B. If not, call your engineer to check the outlet. No engineer? Ask your ECG technician how they eliminate interference. No ECG technician? Find the monitor salesman (often a very helpful person).   (2)

C. If you're monitoring in a ward set-up where interference is a problem, it's often necessary to plug a ground wire into the back of a portable monitor. The other end of this ground wire has an "alligator clip" (it looks like jaws and is capable of biting); you attach this to a water pipe. Try using the radiator if there are no water lines. (1)

12. Find the rate meter. It's like a computer that shows heart rate at all times. See if it's accurate. All you have to do is check the rate on the meter and compare it with the patient's radial pulse. If they are not the same, believe your watch; someone may have fiddled with the rate meter. (2)

13. Find the Low-Rate Alarm. Set it around 50. (2)

14. Find the High-Rate Alarm. Set it about 20 points above the patient's pulse rate. Scratch the electrodes with your finger or have the patient wiggle in bed. How does this affect the ECG pattern? Does it do anything to the counter and alarms? (2)

15. Try the "beeper" (volume) on and off, loud and soft. Do you think that beep-per-beat might bother your patient? (It would me.) (2)

16. Identify any other switch, knob, light, lever, or dial, and try it out. 1 point for each.

Scoring

55—How come YOU aren't writing this?

50—When I have my MI, will you be my nurse?

45—You can do better.

40—You'd better do better.

Below 40—Anything would be better. Try it again.

MONITORING PROBLEMS (*ICC, 4th ed., pp. 79-81*)

The care and understanding of monitors is almost like the care and understanding of children. Experience helps. I'll introduce you to Nurse Old Pro and the nurse she's orienting, Nurse Neo Phyte. Maybe we can learn from their experience.

Suppose we visit them on the night shift. Old Pro is relaxing in front of a console containing 5 flickering monitors. Four of the patients are visible in the open unit and one is a convalescent patient in an adjoining room with only his monitor visible. Pro's eyes constantly scan the monitors in front of her.

Pro: Such a quiet night—I'm afraid you won't see much.

Neo: Oh, look at monitor 1. Is that heart block? Shall I call the doctor?

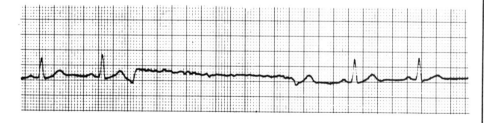

Pro: No, hold on a minute. The first two and the last two complexes are perfectly normal. That squiggly line across the middle doesn't look like it comes from the heart. Notice that sharp V right after the second complex: there's no reason for a pattern to jump up like that. Why don't you go and check the patient's electrodes?

Neo: (checks and returns) One electrode was loose. I taped it down and now he's normal again.

Pro: Too bad we can't patent your method of making people normal. Incidentally, anything on the monitor that is not caused by the heart's action is called an "artifact."

Neo: Oh dear, 2 is going from the top to the bottom of the monitor. That's not right. Does he have a loose electrode, too?

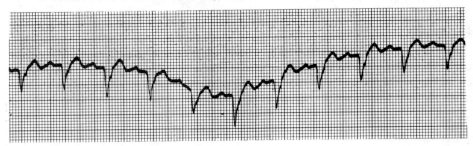

Pro: That's a pattern I like to see. I'll bet you a cup of coffee that he's snoring. That's a respiratory deflection. There are some abnormal things about his pattern, but the "hills and valleys" cycles are just fine. If you want to get rid of them you just reposition the chest electrodes. But let's not awaken him.

Neo: Will I ever learn when to panic?

Pro: (laughing) Of course you will. And I'll tell you a secret. Even the pros panic; we just make good use of that extra adrenalin. Now, don't panic, but I'd like you to check 3. I can still see a regular pattern, but something's going on. I'm just not sure what's causing it.

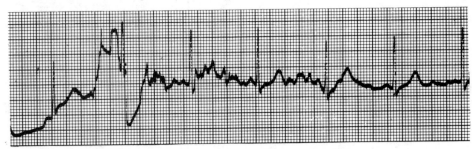

Neo: (returns after several minutes) He was scratching! The electrode jelly makes him itch. I washed his chest off and moved the electrodes a bit.

Pro: That's good. Now what on earth is happening next door on monitor 5? (High-rate alarm sounds.)

Neo: (racing for patient's room) I'll go see!

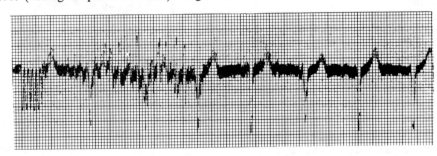

Pro: (to herself) It's electrical interference, but why suddenly in the middle of the night?

Neo: (returns shaking her head) He couldn't sleep, so do you know what he was doing? Shaving with an electric razor!

Pro: Look at those closely spaced lines on his monitor strip. There are actually 60 of them per second. That's 60-cycle electrical interference.

Neo: I don't think I'll count them. By the way, I told the patient that we didn't think it was safe for him to shave with a razor that plugs in the wall. I promised to bring the unit's battery-operated razor in the morning.

Pro: Good. We have to be really careful about shock hazards in the CCU,, especially in patients with transvenous pacemakers.

Neo: Why did the high-rate alarm go off on this patient?

Pro: Look at the strip: the monitor counts all upright lines. It tried to count all the 60-cycle interference, so it exceeded the high-alarm setting. I've got the high set on 110.

Neo: There's so much to learn; how will I know the real thing? I'll probably defibrillate a patient for interference.

Pro: You'll know. I think I'll go get a cup of coffee; I'll be right back. (leaves)

Neo: (A few seconds later the alarm rings on monitor 4.) Oh dear, oh look! That's it—I'm sure its *ventricular fibrillation*! What do I do? I remember—check the patient. (runs to bedside) Mr. Four? Mr. Four? Why don't you answer? No pulse, none. Keep cool. Push the emergency alarm. (Alarm sounds outside the unit.) Get the defibrillator.

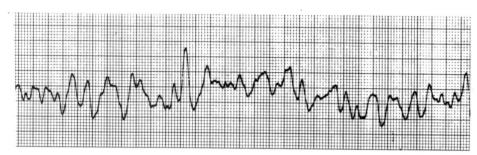

Pro: (races in to answer alarm, looks at patient) Aha, you knew! Good girl. Go ahead, defibrillate him—quickly.

Did you pick up a few ideas on the causes and cures of interference? When you're thoroughly familiar with normal rhythm and arrhythmias, interference will be easy to spot.

COMPUTERIZED ARRHYTHMIA MONITORING
(*ICC, 4th ed., pp. 81-83*)

I remember when the salesperson brought that new-fangled computer monster into our CCU. Those of us who were old-fashioned CCU nurses sniffed skeptically, but soon we were avidly playing with our latest toy. Is computerized arrhythmia monitoring the answer? I don't know. Does your hospital have it? If so, go get acquainted. If not, let's review the principles involved anyway.

Exercise 2

1. A high percentage of serious arrhythmias go undetected in CCUs. (True/False)

> True

2. In theory, a computer can be programmed to recognize _____ ____ _____ and to identify _____.

> normal or
> abnormal arrhythmias

3. The computer's alarm can be programmed so it will "ring" and also _____ _____.

> run a
> rhythm strip

4. The computer can show a continual _____ report and also present an _____ trend.

> status
> hourly

5. Are the computers foolproof? _____

> No! Artifacts fool computers, too.

TELEMETRY (*ICC, 4th ed., pp. 83-85*)

A Candy Striper (high school volunteer) came flying down the hall and nearly crash-landed on the head nurse's desk. "That man—the one with the thing around his neck that makes his heart beat—one of those little wires came off . . . Hurry, he's going to die!"

Just what was she so upset about? The poor panicky Candy Striper misunderstood the function of telemetric monitoring. And so do many other people.

The CCU nurse needs to understand telemetry well enough to be able to apply it and to explain it to the patient, family, and others.

Exercise 3

Let's go over the components of telemetry and see how well you could explain it. Pretend you're talking with your patient, Mr. Kardiak, as you prepare to transfer him out of CCU. Complete the following statements, then check them against my suggestions.

You: Mr. Kardiak, I'm going to put a telemetry set-up on you so that we can continue monitoring you after you move out of CCU.

Mr. Kardiak: You don't say? What are you sticking those things on me for?

You: These electrode pads on your chest _____ _____ _____.

pick up the electrical signals that come from your heart

Mr. Kardiak: Hmm, what do those little wires do?

You: The electrode wires _____ _____ _____.

carry the signals to this little box that you'll wear around your neck

Mr. Kardiak: That thing you're putting around my neck . . . what's it do?

You: This little box that you'll be wearing is a _____.

transmitter

It will _____ _____ _____.

send your heart's pattern back to the nurses' station as radio waves

Mr. Kardiak: How about that! What makes it work?

You: There is a _____ inside this box that keeps it operating.

battery

Mr. Kardiak: Great. What happens to the signals after they reach the nurses' station?

You: There's an antenna out in the hall that sends the waves to a _____ in CCU.

monitor

Mr. Kardiak: Really? You mean, even though I'm out of sight, in the CCU you can still see my heart?

You: That's right. The CCU nurses will _____ _____.

keep a close watch on how your heart behaves

Mr. Kardiak: That's kinda comforting to know.

You: If the _____ or _____ become loose, we'll have to come in and fix them because this will cause too much interference in the pattern that the CCU nurses are seeing. So if we have to bother you in the middle of the night, we're apologizing in advance.

electrodes, wires

Mr. Kardiak: No sweat. I'm used to you folks waking me up.

You: Now, I want to be sure you understand that telemetry only shows up a pattern like an ECG of your heart's activity. It does not _____ _____. So there's no danger if you become unhooked. OK?

control (or affect) how your heart beats

Mr. Kardiak: Yeah, I got that straight. But can I get a shock from this?

You: No, it does not conduct any electricity from the battery to you. So you can't _____.

get a shock from it

(The next day you ask Mr. Kardiak if he has any questions.)

Mr. Kardiak: I sure do. During the night they came in and switched these little things on my chest all around. What were they doing?

You: They changed the position of the electrodes to get a different _____ _____. The pattern they were seeing wasn't clear enough. It's similar to your TV set—sometimes one channel comes in better than the others. I guess you could say that they switched channels on your "TV" to get a clearer picture of your heart.

picture of your heart

The Major Complications of an MI

Chapter 7 of *Intensive Coronary Care*, 4th ed., is tremendously important. It discusses in detail the 5 major complications of an MI. We'll consider these one at a time, using several subsections for each.

HEART FAILURE (*ICC, 4th ed., p. 87*)

Exercise 1

1. A synonym for heart contraction is _____.   systole

2. A synonym for the relaxation period between contractions is _____.   diastole

3. If the heart can't empty completely during systole, some blood _____   remains
   in the ventricles.

4. The remaining blood _____ with subsequent filling of the ven-   interferes
   tricles.

5. Since the ventricles are partly full to begin with, there is an _____ in   increase
   pressure within the chambers during diastole.

6. This increased pressure causes returning blood to back up into the _____   atria
   and _____ system.   venous

7. The heart may compensate for this by _____ its rate and force of   increasing
   contraction.

8. If this compensatory mechanism isn't adequate, the heart begins to _____.   fail

LEFT VENTRICULAR FAILURE (*ICC, 4th ed., pp. 87-89*)

Now we'll see how all this relates to acute myocardial infarction.

Exercise 2

1. In acute myocardial infarction, the _____ ventricle is usually damaged.   left

2. Therefore, the MI may _____ the strength of left ventricular contraction.

weaken or decrease

3. This causes the pumping ability of the left ventricular to _____.

decrease

4. With each stroke (contraction) the weakened, ischemic left ventricle pumps a _____ volume of blood.

reduced or lesser

5. This means that there is a reduction in s_____ v_____.

stroke volume

6. With the heart pumping less volume, its total output _____.

falls

7. Thus we say the _____ falls.

cardiac output

8. Cardiac output = stroke volume × _____ per minute.

beats

9. If the stroke volume is 50 cc/minute and the heart rate is 80 beats/minute, the cardiac output is _____ cc/minute.

4,000 (50 × 80)

10. Two compensatory mechanisms used by the heart to increase cardiac output are _____ and _____ _____ of _____.

tachycardia, increased force contraction

11. The failing left ventricle pumps less blood with each contraction and empties (completely/incompletely).

incompletely

12. The left ventricle pumps blood into the _____ circulation.

systemic

13. Blood returns to the left ventricle from the lungs through the _____ _____ into the left atrium.

pulmonary
veins

14. When returning blood enters the partly full and failing left ventricle, the pressure _____ during diastole.

rises

15. This is known as increased v_____ d_____ p_____.

ventricular diastolic
pressure

16. This increase in left ventricular pressure causes a back pressure in the _____ _____ and in the _____ _____.

left
atrium, pulmonary veins

17. The increased pulmonary venous pressure forces_____ from the capillaries into the lung tissues.

fluid

18. The right ventricle is (often/seldom) affected by acute MI.

seldom

19. Thus, _____ heart failure is not common in MI.

right

20. If it occurs, it is usually the result of_____ ventricular failure.

left

INCIPIENT LEFT VENTRICULAR FAILURE
(*ICC, 4th ed., pp. 89-90*)

Left ventricular failure ranges from the mildest asymptomatic form to the distressingly acute and sometimes fatal pulmonary edema. We begin with incipient left ventricular failure, the mildest type.

Exercise 3

1. The very first stage of impending left ventricular failure is (increased/decreased) pressure in the pulmonary veins.

increased

2. Initially the increased pulmonary venous pressure (does/does not) produce symptoms.

does not

3. Nonetheless, it can be diagnosed by _____.

chest x-ray

4. This is called incipient or _____ left ventricular failure.

subclinical

5. Further pulmonary venous hypertension may force _____ from the capillaries into the tissues surrounding the alveoli of the lungs.

fluid

6. This fluid is called _____ edema. — interstitial

7. Interstitial edema means there is fluid in the tissues _____ _____. — around the alveoli

8. Interstitial edema (does/does not) cause symptoms. — does not

9. But it can be diagnosed on _____. — chest x-ray

10. Thus, one purpose of a chest x-ray in patients with MI is to detect _____ left ventricular failure. — early or incipient

CLINICAL MANIFESTATIONS OF LEFT VENTRICULAR FAILURE (*ICC, 4th ed., pp. 90-91*)

Overt left ventricular failure means that the patient has developed obvious signs and symptoms as a result of the failing heart. Unlike incipient failure, which produces no symptoms and can only be detected by x-ray, overt failure is easily recognized by physical examination.

Exercise 4

1. As pressure continues to increase in the pulmonary capillaries, fluid is forced into the _____, or air cells, of the lungs. — alveoli

2. This is called _____ edema. — alveolar

3. With alveolar edema the patient has the symptom of _____. — dyspnea

4. The cardinal physical sign of alveolar edema is _____. — rales

5. Since mild dyspnea is difficult to observe, you should ask if the patient _____ _____ _____ _____. — feels short of breath

6. Requests by the patient to elevate the head of the bed may indicate the form of dyspnea called _____. — orthopnea

7. When the patient suffers from dyspnea while lying flat, this shortness of breath is termed _____. — orthopnea

8. Normally the heart has two sounds. In left ventricular failure, a _____ sound is often heard. — third

9. This is called a _____ rhythm. — gallop

10. It represents another sign of _____ _____ _____. — left ventricular failure

11. The two most important physical findings of left ventricular failure are _____ and a _____ _____. — rales gallop rhythm

12. General, nonspecific signs of heart failure that a nurse should watch for include: _____, _____, and _____. — tachycardia, sweating, restlessness

Exercise 5

You have never heard a ventricular gallop. How do you identify one? First, listen closely to many normal hearts; get used to the S_1 and S_2 sounds. After you have become familiar with normal heart sounds, read the doctor's notes and listen in during report to discover those patients who have a ventricular gallop. Take your stethoscope to the patient and

1. Listen carefully to the two normal heart sounds; they're called _____ and _____. — S_1 S_2

2. To hear a gallop rhythm, place the (bell/diaphragm) of your stethoscope over the _____ of the heart. — bell apex

61

3. If it's a ventricular gallop rhythm, you will hear an extra sound (before/after) the (first/second) sound.

after
second

4. This is called an _____ sound.

S_3

5. Sometimes you may also hear an extra sound that comes just before S_1. This is an _____ gallop.

atrial

6. Rather than call this a pre-S_1, it is termed an _____ gallop.

S_4

7. S_4 is (more/less) serious than S_3.

less

8. An S_3 indicates _____ of the left ventricle.

dilation

9. Thus an S_3 is a definite sign of _____ _____ _____.

left ventricular failure

PAROXYSMAL NOCTURNAL DYSPNEA

(ICC, 4th ed., pp. 90-91)

I wish that, while you're studying this, you could actually take care of patients with left ventricular failure. Then the words on page 91 of *ICC*, 4th ed., would come alive for you. If you have any patients with this diagnosis, try to spend some time observing them. As a poor secondbest, I'll tell you about two patients I remember. Would you please join me on the night shift of the day this actually happened?

We were only halfway through our CCU course, incompetent, unready, but inescapably there. Cardiac patients seemed to be everywhere, but our CCU wasn't ready yet. In desperation we gathered the patients and emergency supplies into a six-bed ward, a cardiac ward.

"Mr. Kardiak had a quiet evening. No complaints. Asleep by 10." The PM nurse closed the Kardex and went home. The shadows settled down on our makeshift set-up.

Twelve o'clock and all was . . . Was that a small cough? Suddenly Mr. Kardiak launches himself bolt upright in bed, wheezing, choking, clutching his chest, shaking the side rails. He coughs and sneezes and gasps, "Can't breathe—air—window."

I run to his bed, stumbling over the oxygen tank. The pain in my ankle activates my brain. "This oxygen will do you more good than the window. You'll be able to breathe easier with it on," I say as you quickly turn on the tank and together we strap on his mask. "If you sit still, you'll need less air," I tell him. "We'll put the side rails down and help you sit on the edge of the bed if you promise not to run for the window."

You drop the side rail and we support him on the edge of the bed. Even though he's panting and purple, we reassure him, and in a few minutes that seem like hours his dyspnea eases.

Finally, he collapses into sleep and we collapse at our desk. We've just handled our first case of paroxysmal nocturnal dyspnea (PND).

Exercise 6

1. Explain the term *paroxysmal nocturnal dyspnea.*
   Paroxysmal because _____.

   the attack starts suddenly

   Nocturnal because _____.

   it usually occurs at night

   Dyspnea because _____.

   the main symptom is marked shortness of breath

2. Although PND occurs suddenly, the patient has probably had _____ left ventricular failure first.

   incipient

3. If the patient wants to sit up, what should you do? _____

   Let him sit up.

4. Which is the most effective way of giving this patient oxygen? _____

   with a face mask

5. Obviously, the patient is frightened by this terrifying experience. What can you do about this? _____
   _____.

   Talk to him and reassure him that the attack will soon pass.

6. Physical examination during an attack of PND often reveals rales throughout the lungs. This means the patient has developed _____ edema.

alveolar

7. Alveolar edema is a sign of incipient heart failure (True/False).

False

8. Another term for PND is _____.

cardiac asthma

ACUTE PULMONARY EDEMA (*ICC, 4th ed., p. 91*)

Now that you've had a short break, won't you come back to our "Cardiac Ward"? Did I mention we had one empty bed? Well, Dr. Hart is going to remedy that; he's just called from ER. I'm scared: Dr. Hart sounded frantic.

The phone was still warm when he crashed through the door with the stretcher, and with one quick move we transfer his emergency patient to Bed 1. He says, "We'll need oxygen, an IV, morphine, a Foley, a diuretic, and digitalis." Then he whispers, "He's moribund."

I run for the drugs while you help the patient. Our emergency is a miniature Santa Claus: white hair, white mustache, and an adorable goatee. But his beard is covered with a creeping, crawling, bubbling foam, a frothy mucus that pours incessantly out of his nose and mouth and nearly engulfs him. He's coughing, drowning, and is too weak to protest, so you continually wipe the mucus, give him oxygen, and try to talk to him. Meanwhile, Dr. Hart is pawing through our emergency drugs. I plop his favorite IV "intercath" in his hands and tell him, "If you'll start the IV, I'll get the morphine and draw up your diuretic." I'm halfway through when he asks for the digitalis first. "We have Cedilanid, ouabain . . ." He chooses ouabain. I drop onto the bed the syringe I was filling with the diuretic, draw up the digitalis, and at the same time grab a Foley cath set. (You're wrong, I've only got two hands.) Dr. Hart inserts the catheter while I administer the IV drugs slowly.

You leave the mucus-tide to check the BP; you look up, shake your head, and try again. Between pushes on the syringes, I attach the monitor. Dr. Hart swears at the monitor. I'm glad we can't interpret arrhythmias yet. Through all the confusion I hear the soft purr of your voice as you reassure Santa Claus.

Gradually, the pace slows and we all begin to smile. Santa Claus is asleep when we open his chart. Dr. Hart writes his orders, then says, "When I came through that door, I had no idea we could save him." He smiles a good night; we've just helped treat acute pulmonary edema.

Exercise 7

1. The most critical form of acute left ventricular failure is _____ _____.

pulmonary edema

2. This patient had extensive alveolar edema, which causes profound _____ distress.

respiratory

3. See if you can list at least 6 signs or symptoms of acute pulmonary edema.
   1.
   2.
   3.
   4.
   5.
   6.

dyspnea; cyanosis; gurgling respiratory sounds; coughing; frothy, blood-tinged sputum; rapid pulse; sweating; obvious distress

63

TREATMENT OF ACUTE PULMONARY EDEMA
(*ICC, 4th ed., pp. 91-95*)

MECHANISMS AND TREATMENT—LEFT VENTRICULAR FAILURE

III. Myocardial _____

Rx obj. _____

Rx used:

   1. _____

II. Afterload _____

Rx obj. _____

Rx used:

   1. _____

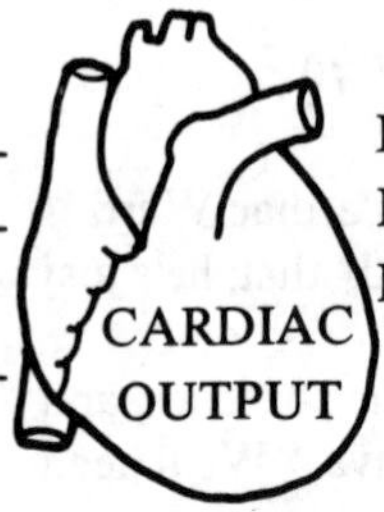

CARDIAC OUTPUT

I. Preload _____

Rx obj. _____

Rx used:

   1. _____

   2. _____

IV. Heart _____

Rx obj. _____

Rx used:

   1. _____

Figure 7.1.

Exercise 8

1. The overall objective in treating left ventricular failure is _____ _____ _____ .

   | increasing cardiac output

2. To do that, we work with the four principle mechanisms in Figure 7.1. Fill in the blanks labeled I-IV in Figure 7.1.

   | I. Volume II. Resistance III. Contractility IV. Rate

3. When the doctor orders drugs or treatments for our patient with acute heart failure, it helps to relate them to the four mechanisms of Figure 7.1. So let's complete the rest of the blanks in that diagram.

MECHANISM I Preload Volume

1. The objective is to (decrease/increase) preload volume, or as the therapy is called, preload volume _____ .

   | decrease
   | reduction

(Write the three words of your last answer in the blank labeled Rx obj. under I in Figure 7.1.)

2. Here we go with the increase/decrease mechanisms again. Put your choice (increases/decreases) in the blanks. Preload volume reduction _____ filling of the left ventricle, _____ pulmonary venous pressure, and thus _____ stroke volume, _____ cardiac output and _____ pulmonary venous congestion.

   | decreases
   | decreases
   | increases, increases
   | decreases

3. Drugs used to increase urinary output and decrease blood volume are _____. (Write your answer in under I, 1. in Figure 7.1.)

   | diuretics

4. Drugs used to dilate or relax peripheral blood vessels are called _____. (Write your answer in under I, 2. in Figure 7.1.)

   | vasodilators

64

5. Vasodilators can dilate the _____ system, the _____ system, or both. | venous, arterial

6. The desired results of the vasodilator, nitroglycerin, would be venous _____ of the blood. | pooling

7. To summarize: in treating left ventricular failure you may give your patients drugs that are classified as _____ or _____ to achieve _____ _____ _____. | diuretics, vasodilators preload volume reduction

MECHANISM II Afterload Resistance

1. The second method of treatment for advanced heart failure is afterload _____. (Write the two words in your answer in the blank labeled Rx. obj. under II in Figure 7.1.) | reduction

2. Treatment of afterload resistance is designed to decrease the _____ against which the heart must pump. | pressure or resistance

3. High arterial pressure (decreases/increases) stroke volume and (decreases/increases) the heart's work. | decreases, increases

4. The doctor might order _____ to reduce ventricular afterload. (Write your answer in under II, 1. in Figure 7.1.) | vasodilators

5. You would watch very carefully for the serious complication of _____ with vasodilator drugs. | hypotension

MECHANISM III Myocardial Contractility

1. The objective of treatment of this mechanism is to _____ _____ _____. (Write the three words of your answer in the blank labeled Rx. obj. under III in Figure 7.1.) | increase myocardial contractility

2. If you can strengthen myocardial contractility, you will (increase/decrease) ventricular emptying, and thus the blood left in the ventricle (residual volume) should (increase/decrease). | increase / decrease

3. This should improve stroke _____ and cardiac _____. | volume, output

4. _____ therapy has long been used for this purpose. (Write your answer in III, 1. in Figure 7.1.) | Digitalis

5. Dangerous complications to watch for with digitalis therapy in acute MIs are _____ and increased energy expenditure of the heart. | arrhythmias

MECHANISM IV Heart Rate

1. Heart rates that are too _____ or too _____ result in decreased cardiac _____. | fast, slow output

2. The objective of the treatment of this mechanism is to _____ the heart _____. (Write the four words of your answer in the blank labeled Rx. obj. under IV in Figure 7.1.) | regulate rate

3. Fast rates don't allow time for the ventricles to _____ and thus decrease _____. | fill volume

4. Slow rates decrease cardiac _____ because of their infrequency. | output

5. Drugs or cardiac _____ may be used to regulate the heart's rate. (Write the two words of your answer in blank IV, 1. in Figure 7.1.) | pacing

Exercise 9

In treating acute pulmonary edema, you must consider the following points.

POINT 1

1. Morphine is used to reduce anxiety and to _____ the brain's respiratory center.

   depress

2. This helps (decrease/increase) the respiratory rate.

   decrease

3. Morphine also decreases preload volume by its _____ effect on peripheral veins.

   vasodilator

POINT 2

1. Alveolar edema (increases/decreases) the available space for air in the lungs.

   decreases

2. Therapy with _____ helps to increase the concentration of oxygen available to the alveoli.

   oxygen

3. The nasal cannula is the (most/least) effective means of administering oxygen.

   least

4. If necessary, oxygen can be given using an _____ machine.

   IPPB

5. In this situation, _____ _____ may be used instead of water as an anti-foaming agent.

   ethyl alcohol

POINT 3

1. _____ are drugs that help the body eliminate excess fluids.

   Diuretics

2. Two rapid-acting IV diuretics are _____ and _____.

   Lasix, Edecrin

3. Their generic names are _____ and _____ _____.

   furosemide, ethacrynic acid

4. Theoretically, they (increase/decrease) elimination of extracellular fluid.

   increase

5. This, in turn, (increases/decreases) the blood volume returning to the heart, which then (increases/decreases) pulmonary venous pressure and reduces edema.

   decreases
   decreases

POINT 4

1. Vasodilators promote "pooling" of the blood and thus _____ preload volume.

   reduce

2. The venous dilator _____ 0.4 to 0.8 mg sublingually can relieve dyspnea in 2 to 3 minutes.

   nitroglycerin

3. The generic name for longer lasting, slower onset nitrates used to decrease pulmonary edema is _____ _____.

   isosorbide dinitrate

4. Two isosorbide dinitrates you might find in your CCU are _____ and _____.

   Isordil
   sorbitrate

5. Two vasodilators that work on both venous and arterial networks are _____ and _____.

   nitroprusside, prazosin

6. Of the four mechanisms, _____ _____ is the most difficult to treat.

   heart rate

7. During vasodilator therapy, we watch patients for the complications of _____ and postural _____.

   headaches, hypotension

POINT 5

1. Digitalis (is/is not) now the cornerstone of the treatment program for left ventricular failure after an MI. | is not

2. Digitalis may be used to improve myocardial_____ if treatment with nitrates and diuretics is ineffective. | contractility

3. Digitalis is most likely to be used after the first_____ days of an MI and will be given by _____ mode. | 4
   intravenous

POINT 6

1. Bronchodilators are used to relieve _____. | bronchospasm

2. The most common bronchodilator is _____ dosage _____-_____ mg given IV. | aminophylline, 250-500

3. Aminophylline's beneficial actions include:_____ bronchioles, _____ cardiac output, and _____ venous pressure. | dilating
   increasing, decreasing

4. Aminophylline's side effects may be _____ and _____. | hypotension
   arrhythmias

5. Suppose Dr. Halforder calls and says: "Give aminophylline 250 mg IV stat and repeat prn." How would you give it?

   Check all correct notations below:

A. undiluted	E. fast push	B and H
B. dilute to 50 cc	F. over 5 minutes	
C. dilute to 100 cc	G. over 10 minutes	
D. in 500 cc D$_5$W	H. over 15 minutes	

   The prn repeat is usually:

A. every 30-60 minutes	C. every 3-4 hours	C
B. every 1-2 hours	D. every 6-8 hours	

POINT 7

1. Rotating tourniquets may be used to_____ venous blood in the extremities. | pool or trap

2. Less frequently, phlebotomy is used to _____ blood and decrease circulating volume. | remove

3. Both help to (increase/decrease) blood volume. | decrease

RIGHT HEART FAILURE (*ICC, 4th ed., pp. 96-97*)

So far we've been talking about the left side of the heart. Now we take a look at the right side. Before starting, go back and review Fig. 7.1 in *ICC,* 4th ed. Try to imagine a force or pressure pushing the blood backwards through the left heart, the lungs, and the right heart. Oversimplified, yes, but understandable.

Exercise 10

1. After an MI, (left/right) heart failure is most common. | left

2. Left heart failure causes pulmonary venous pressure to _____. | rise

3. So when the right heart tries to empty, it meets increased pressure in the pulmonary _____. | circulation

4. Therefore, pulmonary artery pressure also _____.

  rises

5. The right ventricle then (does/does not) empty completely.

  does not

6. Then blood entering the right atrium meets (increased/decreased) pressure.

  increased

7. This causes _____ back pressure within the entire peripheral venous system.

  increased

8. This is called_____ heart failure because the venous system is overloaded.

  congestive

Exercise 11

The theory just discussed is called *backward heart failure*, but as *ICC*, 4th ed., points out on page 96, right heart failure may not always be so simple. An alternative theory is called forward heart failure. It acknowledges that:

1. In congestive heart failure, there may be inadequate blood flow to the _____.

  kidneys

2. This affects _____ function and stimulates the production of certain _____.

  renal hormones

3. These chemical substances cause _____ and _____ to be retained in the body.

  sodium, water

4. Probably both _____ and _____ heart failure exist together.

  backward, forward

Exercise 12

Now we'll consider the symptoms seen in a patient with right heart failure. Remember, now we're looking at a problem that is not just pulmonary, but systemic as well.

1. Overloading of the venous system causes (increased/decreased) venous pressure.

  increased

2. An early sign of overloading in the venous system is_____ of the neck veins.

  distention

3. To be significant, the distention must be visible when the patient is (in a flat position/sitting up).

  sitting up

4. Increased venous pressure forces fluid from the capillaries into the _____ tissues.

  subcutaneous

5. This fluid usually collects in the _____ parts of the body.

  dependent or lowest

6. Thus it is called _____ _____.

  dependent edema

7. Another form of peripheral edema is swelling of the _____ or _____.

  feet, legs

8. At bed rest, this edema may be found on the patient's _____.

  back

9. When edema is present throughout the entire body, it is called _____.

  anasarca

10. Edema that collects between the layers of lining in the lungs is called a_____ _____.

  pleural effusion

11. Edema in the abdominal cavity is called _____.

  ascites

12. Suspect pleural effusion if, as you listen to a patient's lungs with a stethoscope, you note _____ or _____ breath sounds.

  diminished, absent

13. Pain or discomfort in the right upper abdomen may indicate edema of the _____, also due to venous distention.

  liver

14. Other symptoms that may accompany engorgement of the liver are _____ and _____.

  anorexia nausea

15. To detect an engorged liver, use the _____ _____ test.

  hepatojugular reflux

16. Apply pressure over the (left/right) upper quadrant of the abdomen. | right

17. This applies pressure over the _____ and increases venous return to the heart. | liver

18. A positive sign is _____ _____ distention, indicating the _____ _____ cannot accommodate the increased blood flow from the liver. | neck vein, right heart

TREATMENT OF RIGHT HEART FAILURE
(*ICC, 4th ed., pp. 97-99*)

Exercise 13

1. Treatment of right heart failure is aimed at promoting the excretion of _____ and _____. | water / salt

2. Another aim is to improve cardiac _____. | output or performance

3. Providing _____ is one of the most effective ways a nurse can reduce the cardiac workload. | rest

4. A low-sodium diet may permit only _____ mg sodium per day. (Explaining the reasons for this diet may help your patient tolerate it better.) | 1000

5. Sodium restriction is essential in order to decrease the circulating blood _____. | volume

6. In addition to rest and sodium restrictions, _____ are important in the treatment of right heart failure. | diuretics

7. Sodium and water excretion can be increased by the use of _____ drugs. | diuretic

8. Most diuretics work on the _____ of the kidneys. | tubules

9. They prevent the tubules from returning some of the _____ and _____ to the body. | water, salt

10. Thus, the urinary output of _____ and _____ is increased. | water, salt

11. Diuretics also increase excretion of _____. | potassium

12. Low serum potassium is called _____. | hypokalemia

13. Hypokalemia can increase myocardial _____. | irritability

14. Increased myocardial irritability can lead to serious _____. | arrhythmias

15. What signs and symptoms of hypokalemia would you watch for in any patient on a diuretic? _____ | lassitude, anorexia, confusion, decreased urinary output

16. Patients on diuretics will often receive oral or IV _____. | potassium

17. Patients on a restricted sodium diet, with increased sodium loss due to diuresis, may need to have their fluids (increased/restricted). | restricted

18. High fluid intake under these conditions may result in _____ _____. | hyponatremia (low-salt syndrome)

19. After the acute phase of an MI, if other therapies are inadequate, _____ therapy may be used. | digitalis

20. Also used in congestive heart failure if other therapies are inadequate are _____ to decrease afterload resistance. | vasodilators

Exercise 14

The more you can learn about drugs and their actions *now*, the easier it will be when we get to the chapter on drugs. First, let's do some matching of generic and trade names, because you'll inevitably run into some of these. Place the correct number of the "trade" or "brand" name in front of the generic name

Generic		Trade	
_____ Sodium nitroprusside		1. Apresoline	5
_____ Captopril		2. Isordil	3
_____ Isosorbide dinitrate		3. Capoten	4
_____ Isosorbide dinitrate		4. Sorbitrate	2
_____ Hydralazine		5. Nipride	1
_____ Minoxidil		6. Loniten	6
_____ Phentolamine		7. Regitine	7

Exercise 15: Diuretic ABCDs

Match the letters, *A, B, C,* and *D* with the correct statements. More than one letter may be required for some statements.

A—Thiazides   C—Aldosterone antagonists
B—Lasix or Edecrin   D—Triamterene

_____ 1. Highest potency		B
_____ 2. Next highest potency		A
_____ 3. Fastest acting		B
_____ 4. Acts in 2-5 days		C
_____ 5. Acts within 2 hours		A
_____ 6. Blocks reabsorption of sodium in tubules		A, B
_____ 7. Acts against the hormone that causes the body to retain salt		C
_____ 8. Usually given as IV		B
_____ 9. Does not cause hypokalemia		D
_____ 10. Potassium therapy nearly always required		B
_____ 11. Aldactone is an example		C
_____ 12. Dyrenium is another name for it		D
_____ 13. Ethacrynic acid is another name for _____		B, Edecrin
_____ 14. Hydrochlorothiazide is one example of this diuretic		A
_____ 15. Furosemide is another name for _____		B, Lasix

NURSING CARE IN ACUTE HEART FAILURE
(*ICC, 4th ed., pp. 99-101*)

Shall we apply what you've just learned? Let's take the 3 PM report on Mr. Kardiak in CCU.

"Mr. Kardiak has been in normal sinus rhythm, rate around 88. At 2 PM his rate was 94. No arrhythmias noted. His lungs show some rales in the left posterior base. Respiratory rate 12-18. His neck veins are not distended. Hepatojugular reflux negative. He has seemed a little tired and lethargic today; however, the night shift reported he slept poorly, so maybe that explains it."

The day shift trots off to a ballgame or a concert, and you put away thoughts of your morning tennis game or jam making and prepare for a busy evening in CCU. Because Mr. Kardiak is doing so well, you assign him to another nurse. It's 8 PM before you have time to review his vital signs sheet. This is what you note:

4 PM: 99—98—18
6 PM: 99^2—102—20
8 PM: 99^2—112—26

Exercise 16

Grabbing your favorite red stethoscope, you head for his bedside.

1. Before you pounce on Mr. Kardiak with your cold stethoscope, you
   (Choose all the appropriate answers.)
   A. Make small talk.
   B. Introduce yourself.
   C. Ask if he feels weak and fatigued.
   D. Ask how he feels.
   E. Ask if he feels different from yesterday or this morning.
   F. Explain that you want to listen to his heart and lungs.   B, D, E, F

Answers and Comments

A. You don't have time for small talk.
C. A direct question like this plants the idea and may shape the patient's response.

Don't put words in his mouth. Ask general questions and then follow them up with more specific questions.

2. Now ask Mr. Kardiak to sit up and let's listen to:

   A. His lungs for _____.   rales

   B. His heart for _____ _____ .   gallop rhythm

   While you're listening you also note:

   C. Skin in general for _____ .   cyanosis

   D. Sacral area for _____ .   edema

   E. Neck for _____ _____ .   distended veins

3. Finished? Let him lie back and then check the following:

   A. _____ _____ quadrant of the abdomen.   Right upper

   B. You're checking for _____ _____ .   liver enlargement

   C. You press firmly in and up (under the rib cage) to check for _____ hepatojugular
      _____.   reflux

   D. While pressing you watch the _____ _____ .   neck veins

   E. If they fill and stand out, it's a (positive/negative) sign.   positive

   F. Which, in our way of looking at things, is (good/bad).   bad

Now that you've finished, you have noted the following:

   • A sweating, tired, lethargic patient
   • Rales on both sides
   • S₃ gallop
   • Distended neck veins at a 45° sitting angle
   • Positive hepatojugular reflux

Would you call the doctor away from his favorite baseball game?   Yes; sorry about that, Dr. Hart.

Exercise 17

Mr. Kardiak improved. Now it's several days later and suddenly he's in trouble again. He's gasping, gurgling, and coughing up bubbly, bloody mucus. He's struggling frantically for breath and is drenched with perspiration.

1. Mr. Kardiak appears to have_____ _____ _____ .

2. You can do three things instantly and simultaneously.

3. While you're putting the oxygen mask on, try to _____ him that oxygen will help his breathing.

71

4. Three drugs the doctor may order immediately are _____, _____ _____ , and a _____ .

5. One thing you might do if the doctor isn't immediately available is to _____ _____ _____ .

6. You're going to watch the monitor closely for _____ on this patient.

7. Ask the doctor if he'd like to have _____ _____ _____ drawn.

Answers and Comments

1. *Acute pulmonary edema.*

2. *Help the patient to a sitting position in bed, give him oxygen,* and *call the doctor.* (Obviously you need 4 hands or else a helper.) At this point some patients fight the oxygen mask or insist that no air is coming out of it. Reassurance, turning the oxygen up temporarily so they can feel it, letting them hold the mask—sometimes these things help.

3. *Reassure* the patient. Many patients cry, "Let me get to a window for some air!" It may help to reassure them that oxygen will do them more good and that scrambling around will only increase their air-hunger.

4. *Morphine, digitalis,* and a *diuretic.* All will probably be given IV.

5. *Apply rotating tourniquets.* They help trap blood in the extremities and reduce the load on the heart and lungs. Most hospitals have their own procedure for the times and rotation of the tourniquets. One more thought: an IV in the wrist doesn't run well with a tourniquet on the arm above it, so generally only 3 tourniquets are used when an IV is running.

6. *Arrhythmias.* There is an especially high risk of arrhythmias developing when oxygenation is inadequate.

7. *Arterial blood gases* are frequently ordered.

Exercise 18

When the crisis is over, the doctor goes home, but you still have a vital role at the bedside. If you know the reasons for your actions, nursing is more interesting. So try answering these questions, and then check your answers against the discussion that follows:

1. Why would you measure the urine output on this patient every 30 minutes?

2. Why should you carefully record intake on Mr. Kardiak?

3. Why might the doctor order a sodium-restricted diet?

4. Mr. Kardiak is given digitalis. Why would you watch his monitor closely?

5. Mr. Kardiak is also on diuretics. Why do you check his lab reports?

6. Why would you be concerned if hypokalemia is present?

7. Why would you examine Mr. Kardiak carefully at least twice a shift?

Answers and Comments

1. Improved kidney function leads to increased urinary output—a sign that therapy is working. This is no time to say, "I guess there's more urine in his Foley bag." Know down to the last cc what the output is. Further drug and IV therapy often hinges on exactly what the urine output is.

2. Overloading this patient with IV fluids is just as destructive as a heavy spring rain on a dammed-up mountain stream. On the other hand, a high or normal fluid intake can

lead to hyponatremia in a patient who is on diuretics and a sodium-restricted diet. Keep an hourly tab on his intake and output, and know what kind of deficit between the two his doctor feels is tolerable. Call the doctor promptly when the difference between intake and output goes beyond the tolerable range.

3. Sodium-restricted diets are used to decrease salt and fluid retention. Patients hate these diets! Explain the reasons, but don't argue with them about how wretched their food tastes without salt. If you can, provide them with an assortment of salt substitutes; then encourage the patient to conduct his own experiment and find out which brand he likes best. (Remind them to use the substitutes sparingly at first.) Also, ask your diet kitchen to provide a slice of lemon on every tray; some patients prefer it to salt substitutes.

4. Digitalis can cause serious arrhythmias if the dosage is excessive. The amount of digitalis required varies with each patient. You must watch the monitor and the patient for signs of overdose (toxicity). What signs? You'll study arrhythmias beginning with Chapter 10, and you'll see the frequent notation, "May be caused by digitalis." The patient? Watch for nausea, vomiting, diarrhea, headaches, and the patient who says, "Something's wrong with my eyes—I see funny colors." (Green and yellow seem to be popular.)

5. Check lab slips carefully for hypokalemia—low potassium. In fact, check lab slips for everything. The studies are done to help the doctor and you in taking care of the patient.

6. Hypokalemia predisposes to arrhythmias. The poor patient: decreased oxygenation and electrolyte imbalance can cause arrhythmias; diuretics cause hypokalemia, which causes arrhythmias. Everything is against him. He really needs an alert nurse to detect and treat these problems.

7. Mr. Kardiak's progress can be monitored by a thorough, careful nursing assessment.

CARDIOGENIC SHOCK (*ICC, 4th ed., pp. 101-103*)

Cardiogenic shock is a terrible killer. In many hospitals, at least 8 out of 10 patients with cardiogenic shock die. If we only knew for certain what causes cardiogenic shock and exactly how it progresses, perhaps we could treat it effectively. Unfortunately, we don't and we can't. Detecting the earliest signs of cardiogenic shock is currently our only approach, but it is not a real solution. However, if you are vigilant, your patient might be one of the lucky ones who survives. Our discussion begins with some familiar phrases: *inadequate perfusion, stroke volume*, and *cardiac output*.

Exercise 19

1. When the left ventricle pumps out less blood at each stroke, there is a decrease in _____ _____.

   stroke volume

2. If stroke volume decreases markedly, _____ _____ will also decrease.

   cardiac output

3. In cardiogenic shock, cardiac output is severely _____.

   decreased

4. Decreased cardiac output causes a _____ in arterial blood pressure.

   decrease

5. It also results in inadequate _____ of vital organs.

   perfusion

6. Cells in the brain, the heart, and other vital organs then suffer from _____ _____ and _____.

   inadequate oxygen, ischemia

7. This decrease in cardiac output may result from the _____ _____ caused by the infarction.

   muscle damage

8. Cardiogenic shock develops because the damaged _____ _____ is unable to maintain an adequate _____ _____.

   left ventricle
   cardiac output

THE COURSE OF CARDIOGENIC SHOCK
(ICC, 4th ed., pp. 101-102)

Your patient is in trouble because his heart can't put out enough blood to supply the needs of the body. What happens next?

Exercise 20

1. The body may compensate for decreased cardiac output by constricting peripheral _____ .   arterioles

2. This peripheral vasoconstriction tends to divert more blood internally to _____ _____ .   vital organs

3. Inadequate perfusion of vital organs can lead to cellular _____ .   death

4. Or inadequate perfusion may damage certain _____ systems.   enzyme

5. In the last stages of cardiogenic shock, blood vessels dilate and the circulation _____ .   collapses

6. When this happens, cardiogenic shock is termed_____ shock. irreversible

7. With irreversible shock, _____ is inevitable.   death

MANIFESTATIONS OF CARDIOGENIC SHOCK
(ICC, 4th ed., pp. 102-103)

Do you believe you have a "sixth sense"? Well, coupled with keen nursing observation, I might believe it. Have you ever said, "I've got a funny feeling about that patient. He's restless and he seems different"? Is this intuition, or are you detecting the first signs of cardiogenic shock?

Exercise 21

1. Decreased perfusion to the brain often causes _____ changes.   mental

2. What are the first signs of this? _____ and _____ .   Apathy, lassitude

3. Inadequate perfusion of the kidneys causes decreased _____ _____ .   urinary volume

4. If the urinary output falls below _____ cc/hour, be suspicious of decreased cardiac output.   60

5. If the output decreases each hour, what should you do? _____ _____ _____ .   Tell the doctor

6. Decreased urinary output is called _____ .   oliguria

7. Urinary output of less than _____ cc/hour is usually a bad sign.   20

8. No output, that is, _____ , is ominous.   anuria

9. In cardiogenic shock the blood pressure_____ as a result of decreased cardiac output.   falls

10. All patients with hypotension have cardiogenic shock. (True/False)   False

11. The numerical difference between systolic and diastolic blood pressure is called the _____ _____ .   pulse pressure

12. In cardiogenic shock the pulse pressure is _____ .   reduced

13. Because of peripheral vasoconstriction, the patient's skin becomes _____ and _____ .   cold pale

14. At the same time, stimulation of the central nervous system causes the skin to be _____ or _____ .   wet, clammy

15. The 4 classical signs of cardiogenic shock are _____,
    _____, _____, and _____
    _____.

mental changes oliguria, hypotension, cold, moist skin

LACTIC ACIDOSIS (*ICC, 4th ed., p. 103*)

In addition to the hemodynamic effects of cardiogenic shock, there are also profound changes in cellular metabolism. The following exercise reviews these.

Exercise 22

1. Normal cellular metabolism utilizing oxygen is called _____ metabolism.

aerobic

2. The end product of aerobic metabolism is _____ acid.

carbonic

3. The body excretes carbonic acid through the lungs as _____ _____ .

carbon dioxide

4. In cardiogenic shock there is not enough oxygen for_____ metabolism.

aerobic

5. Therefore the body turns to _____ metabolism to preserve cellular life.

anaerobic

6. Anaerobic metabolism produces _____ acid.

lactic

7. The body can't get rid of lactic acid through the lungs or kidneys so it builds up in the _____ .

blood

8. This creates a condition called _____ _____ .

lactic acidosis

9. Body _____ cannot live in an acidotic environment.

cells or tissues

10. Also, in the presence of acidosis, fatal _____ may occur.

arrhythmias

11. Therefore, acidosis cannot be tolerated and _____ must be used to combat it.

alkalis

CARDIOGENIC SHOCK: RECOGNITION AND MEASUREMENTS (*ICC, 4th ed., pp. 103-107*)

Exercise 23: Early Recognition of Cardiogenic Shock

In Goodolefashionedhometown Hospital, patient care is given by nurse's aides. The one RN in charge visits each patient at the beginning and end of the shift (if she has time). Vital signs are checked by the nurse's aide at the beginning of the shift and repeated only if the early check is abnormal. Eight-hour intake and outputs are done as ordered on certain patients.

The early-shift check on Mr. T.O.O. Late revealed: 99—80—18, 110/70; there was no late-shift recheck. Head Nurse, Ms. Ova Work, makes a hurried final rounds 10 minutes before report. She finds Mr. T.O.O. Late difficult to arouse, apathetic, and his skin cold and clammy to the touch. She goes off in search of a blood pressure cuff and stethoscope (a difficult feat because the nurse's aides hide them to prevent other floors from borrowing them). Because it's report time, she asks the nurse's aide to find the equipment and check Mr. T.O.O. Late.

The aid interrupts report: "His BP is 84/66."
Ms. Ova Work asks: "And his pulse?"
"You didn't ask me to take that," the aide replies.
A disgusted aide tromps off, checks his pulse, and interrupts report again: "His pulse is 114."

Ms. Ova Work has that sinking feeling as she asks: "How's his urine output been?"
"Well, he had something like 250 cc out."
"Do you know if his output diminished near the end of the shift?"

"No, but come to think of it, it seems to me that most of that was in his bag earlier this morning. Maybe his Foley's plugged? Want me to irrigate it?"

You get the picture, I'm sure. Early recognition of cardiogenic shock is crucial. But it requires planned, repeated checks by a knowledgeable nurse.

Exercise 24: Hemodynamic and Physiological Measurements

1. Usual blood pressure measurements as taken with a cuff and stethoscope (do/do not) always reflect cardiogenic shock.

   do not

2. _____ _____ pressure measurements are more accurate.

   Direct arterial

3. To directly measure arterial pressure, an intraarterial catheter is usually inserted in the _____ artery.

   radial

4. A Foley catheter (is/is not) necessary in the treatment of shock.

   is

5. Urinary output should be measured every _____ minutes.

   30

6. Arterial _____ _____ are drawn to measure PO_2, PCO_2, and pH.

   blood gases

7. Pressure in the right atrium and the superior vena cava can be measured using a _____ _____ _____ catheter.

   central venous pressure

8. Normal CVP ranges from _____ to _____ cm H_2O.

   5, 10

9. CVP measures the ability of the (right/left/neither) ventricle to handle venous return.

   right

10. The relationship between right and left ventricular pressure (is/is not) constant.

   is not

11. CVPs above 15-20 cm H_2O may indicate _____ _____ .

   cardiogenic shock

Exercise 25: Pulmonary Artery Pressure

Foley catheters don't bother you a bit, right? Then come on and try the Swan-Ganz catheter. Start with the same principle of 2 lumens—one to inflate a balloon and one to handle the business of measuring. (Some special Swan-Ganz catheters have 4 lumens and allow you to take 2 extra measurements; we'll stick to the 2-lumen variety in this discussion.)

Swan-Ganz terminology glitters with initialed frenzy: LVEDP, PAP, PWP, PCWP, etc. Let's take it step by step and make some sense out of it.

1. In a patient with impaired cardiac function, we'd really like to measure (and assist) the performance of the (right/left) ventricle.

   left

2. This patient's left ventricle (can/cannot) pump out all the blood it receives with each beat.

   cannot

3. Thus the volume and pressure in the left ventricle is greater than normal at the end of the filling period, which is during _____ .

   diastole

4. Using some of those glorious initials, we say there is an increase in _____ .

   LVEDP

5. Make sure you've got that; spell it out: _____ _____ _____ _____ .

   left ventricular end-diastolic pressure

6. Can we measure LVEDP directly? (Yes/No)

   Yes, but not very easily

76

7. It's safer and easier to pass a catheter into the right side of the heart; how far can it go? _____ _____ .

To the pulmonary arterial branches

8. Here we can record a pressure that reflects the force of contraction of the right ventricle, the resistance in the pulmonary arteries, and the back pressure the left atrium meets as it empties into the left ventricle. Together these groups are referred to as the _____ . _____ _____ .

pulmonary artery pressure (PAP)

9. Now, if we could reduce the number of factors we're measuring, we'd have a clearer picture. Can we do that? (Yes/No)

Yes

10. Inflate the balloon of the Swan-Ganz catheter (it's located 1 mm from the tip of the catheter) and we block out the influence of _____ _____ contraction on the reading.

right ventricular

11. By inflating the balloon, the pressure reading more accurately reflects pulmonary pressure and _____ atrial events.

left

12. Let's back up: The left ventricle does not empty completely, so the left _____ meets with resistance and higher pressure when it tries to empty into the left ventricle.

atrium

13. Therefore, when the blood tries to empty into the _____ _____ , the pulmonary circulation meets with increased pressure.

left atrium

14. The pressure and congestion in the pulmonary veins backs up into the pulmonary _____ .

capillaries

15. An inflated, balloon-tipped catheter inserted into the pulmonary artery records the pressure we call _____ _____ _____ _____ .

pulmonary capillary wedge pressure (PCWP)

16. Is it possible to continuously monitor PCWP by leaving the inflated balloon in the artery? Why or why not?

No. That would cause a pulmonary embolus to develop.

17. So, with the balloon *deflated*, you measure _____ _____ _____ .

pulmonary artery pressure (PAP)

18. Then inflate the balloon (with about 1.5 ml air) and measure the _____ .

PCWP

19. What next?

Deflate the balloon.

20. Usually, there (is/is not) a close correlation between PAP and PCWP.

is

SWAN-GANZ PRESSURE RECORDINGS
(*ICC, 4th ed., pp. 104-105*) (plus illustration pages)

A detailed description of how to insert and maintain a Swan-Ganz catheter is beyond the scope of this book. You can obtain more information from the literature distributed by the manufacturers of the equipment. Also check the indexes of the nursing magazines; there have been many articles (including excellent pictorial ones) in the past few years.

However, we can use the diagrams shown here to follow the route of the Swan-Ganz catheter through the heart as well as look at some pressure recordings similar to those you will see. The recordings can be seen on your patient's pressure monitor as the doctor advances the catheter into the desired position.

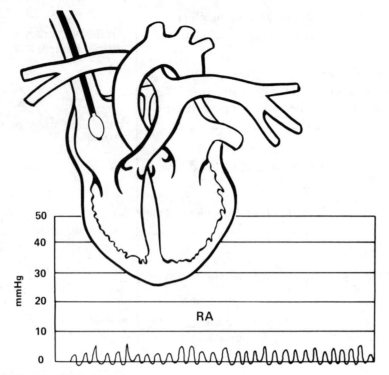

Figure 7.2A. The Right Atrium.

The normal right atrium is pretty much a low-pressure system. The pressure recordings seen on the monitor are minimal, similar to this and below 10 mm Hg.

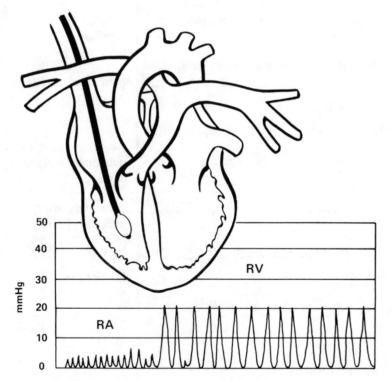

Figure 7.2B. The Right Ventricle.

The inflated balloon helps the catheter to float as it is advanced into the right ventricle. According to Meltzer *et al.*, the normal right ventricular pressure is 20/5. (Compare that to the systemic pressure of 130/70.)

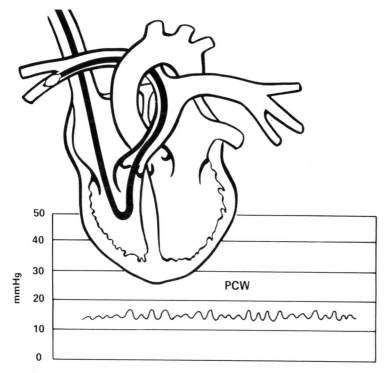

Figure 7.3A. Pulmonary Capillary Wedge Pressure.

The catheter, with balloon inflated, is advanced until it wedges in a small branch of the pulmonary artery. Normal capillary wedge pressure ranges from 5-12 mm Hg.

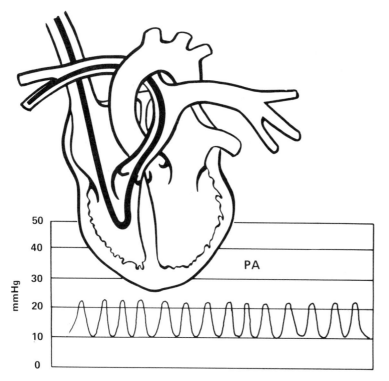

Figure 7.3B. Pulmonary Artery Pressure.

With the balloon deflated the normal PAP is 25/10. Diastolic pressure is used to assess left ventricular function.

Exercise 26

Because these pressure readings are new to many of us, perhaps we need to review them again. Remember that normal varies for individuals and according to the accuracy of the measurements.

1. CVP readings are measured by a (H_2O/Hg) manometer.

H_2O

2. The normal CVP range is _____ to _____ .

5, 10 mm H_2O

3. CVP measures venous pressure in the _____ _____ _____ and reflects back pressure from the _____ _____ .

superior vena cava
right atrium

4. Swan-Ganz pressures are measured in mm (H_2O/Hg).

Hg

5. Normal right atrial pressures range from 12 mm during_____ to 3 mm during _____ .

systole
diastole

6. The normal PAP is _____ systolic and _____ diastolic.

25, 10

7. The (systolic/diastolic) pressure in the pulmonary artery is used to assess left ventricular function.

diastolic

8. Diastolic PAP above _____ may indicate that the left ventricle is not emptying completely.

12

9. PCWP is measured with the balloon _____ .

inflated

10. PCWP of _____ to _____ is considered normal.

5, 12

11. If the PCWP rises above _____ , it may indicate that the left ventricle is not emptying completely.

12

CARDIAC OUTPUT (ICC, 4th ed., p. 104)

Exercise 27

1. Cardiac output can be monitored using a cold saline solution; this is called the _____ method.

thermodilution

2. This is done through a modified _____ catheter.

Swan-Ganz

3. The catheter has a built-in electrode called a_____ that detects temperature changes.

thermister

4. The catheter is floated into the _____ _____ .

pulmonary artery

5. When cold saline is injected, it goes out the lumen that is positioned in the right _____ or the _____ _____ .

atrium, vena cava

6. This causes a temperature change that the thermister measures in the _____ _____ .

pulmonary artery

7. A (greater/lesser) temperature change in the pulmonary artery reflects a decreased cardiac output.

greater

8. Less of a temperature change reflects a (higher/lower) cardiac output.

higher

9. These measurements of cardiac output are used to evaluate the effectiveness of _____ .

treatment

TREATMENT OF CARDIOGENIC SHOCK
(ICC, 4th ed., pp. 107-110)

Exercise 28: Cardiogenic Shock and Supportive Therapy

We really got carried away with physiological measurements, didn't we? Now, if you've finished taking ABP, UO, ABG, CVP, PAP, and PCWP, don't you think it's time we *treat* the poor cardiogenic shock patient (or is it the nurse who requires treatment by now)?

1. Cardiogenic shock must be treated _____ for best results.

   immediately

2. Supportive therapy includes the administration of _____ , the relief of _____ , and the correction of _____ .

   oxygen
   pain, acidosis

3. Arterial blood gases (should/should not) be performed while the patient is on oxygen.

   should

4. PO$_2$ below _____ indicates respiratory assistance may be needed.

   75

5. Pain should be relieved with (oral/IM/IV) medication.

   IV

6. Why that route?

   Absorption decreases with poor circulation.

7. As you recall, during cardiogenic shock the body reverts to _____ metabolism because of poor perfusion.

   anaerobic

8. An end product of anaerobic metabolism is _____ .

   lactic acid

9. Lactic acidosis may lead to lethal cardiac _____ .

   arrhythmias

10. Lactic acidosis is treated with _____ _____ .

    sodium bicarbonate

11. Complete your own pH scale below. Fill in the normal pH range and insert the terms *acidosis* and *alkalosis* under the scale in the correct places.

    Normal pH range = _____ to _____
    7.30   7.35   7.40   7.45   7.50

    7.35 to 7.45

    1. _____   2. _____

    1. acidosis
    2. alkalosis

12. pH values below _____ indicate acidosis.

    7.35

Exercise 29: Cardiogenic Shock and Specific Treatment

About 10% of the cardiogenic shock patients respond to plasma volume expansion. Identification and treatment of this small group are worthwhile. How can you identify those few patients who might respond to volume expansion?

1. When we speak of patients with a dangerously depleted circulating plasma volume, we say they are _____ . (Nurses often say they're dried out like prunes, but that's not the answer!)

   hypovolemic

2. Consider the causes of this condition in a patient with severe MI: he loses fluids due to _____ and _____ .

   vomiting, diaphoresis

3. Also, he's probably being treated with _____ to increase fluid output.

   diuretics

4. We're afraid of overloading a weak heart so we curtail IV intake. The patient also suffers from _____ , so he eats and drinks little.

   anorexia

5. Unless we're careful we'll end up with a low _____ volume.

   plasma

6. CVP and PAP on this patient would be (low/normal/high).

   low or normal

7. The typical cardiogenic shock patient has (low/normal/high) CVP and PAP readings.

   high

8. With a low CVP or PAP, a trial _____ _____ can be used to see if blood pressure and urine output increase.

   fluid loading

9. In this situation, you might expect an order to administer 200 cc D$_5$W in _____ minutes.

   10

81

10. If the patient responds to volume expansion, his prognosis is (poor/good).   good

Exercise 30: Drug Therapy

1. Inotropic drugs are used to _____ the pumping ability of the heart.   strengthen

2. Inotropic drugs also (decrease/increase) myocardial oxygen consumption.   increase

3. This effect is (dangerous/desirable).   dangerous

4. Levarterenol (trade name: _____) and dopamine (trade name: _____) are 2 inotropic drugs frequently used.   Levophed Inotropin

5. Another inotropic drug is dobutamide or trade name: _____ .   Dobutrex

6. During inotropic drug therapy, you'd be satisfied if the patient had a systolic pressure of _____ to _____ .   90, 100 mm Hg

7. As the drugs are being administered, you watch the monitor for _____.   arrhythmias

8. You expect the drugs to act within (10-30 minutes/1-2 hours/3-6 hours).   1-2 hours

9. _____ , the opposite of vasopressor drugs, may be tried on a limited number of patients suffering from cardiogenic shock.   Vasodilators

10. The theory of vasodilator therapy is that there is so much peripheral vasoconstriction that the left ventricle suffers because _____ _____ .   it has to pump against such strong resistance

11. Thus, _____ drugs may be used to decrease peripheral resistance.   vasodilator

12. The disadvantage is that vasodilators (lower/raise) blood pressure.   lower

13. Vasodilators should *not* be used if a patient's systolic pressure is below_____.   100 mm Hg

14. Drugs or pacing may be used to maintain a heart rate of between _____ and _____ beats/min.   60 100

Exercise 31: Mechanical Assistance

Perhaps you're tired of filling in the blanks. Let's try a few straightforward questions.

1. What does the survival of the cardiogenic shock patient finally depend on (i.e., what physiological basis)?

2. Although inotropic drugs may help, they also have what serious side effects?

3. If cardiogenic shock patients do not respond to drug therapy, what procedure should be considered next?

Answers

1. The amount of oxygen available to the myocardium and the degree of tissue perfusion.

2. Inotropic drugs increase myocardial oxygen consumption; thus the heart requires more oxygen than before.

3. Mechanical assistance or Intraaortic Balloon Pump (IABP).

Exercise 32: The Intraaortic Balloon Pump

1. Blood enters the coronary arteries during (systole/diastole).   diastole

2. The blood supply to the coronary arteries is from the _____ .   aorta

3. An increase in aortic pressure during diastole might (decrease/increase) the filling of the coronary arteries.   increase

82

4. The IABP does this by inserting and inflating a balloon in the aorta at the onset of (systole/diastole).

    diastole

5. The balloon catheter is inserted in the aorta through the _____ artery.

    femoral

6. A pump inflates the balloon with _____ at the onset of diastole.

    helium

7. The pump deflates the balloon _____ _____ _____ to decrease resistance when the heart contracts.

    just before systole

8. The sudden decrease in aortic pressure (reduces/increases) the workload of the left ventricle.

    reduces

9. The IABP is syncronized with (respirations/heartbeat).

    heartbeat

10. It has proven very difficult to _____ patients away from IABP.

    wean

Exercise 33

List 4 identifying features of cardiogenic shock:

1.

    Low blood pressure, especially when there is narrowed pulse pressure

2.

    Mental confusion, apathy, anxiety, or lethargy

3.

    Decreasing urinary output

4.

    Cold, clammy skin

Exercise 34

You've just checked your patient, Mr. Kardiak. He has all of those signs you've just listed and a BP of 78/56. Imagine yourself in a small hospital ICU—no house doctors. While your assistant calls Dr. Hart, what are you going to do? List the steps you'd take while the doctor is being called. (Answers follow this exercise.)

1.

2.

3.

4.

5.

6.

7.

Answers

1. Place Mr. Kardiak supine with a pillow under his head. No Trendelenburg position, please!

2. Give him oxygen per mask at 8-10 liters.

3. If he's in pain, give him morphine, 5 mg IV (if ordered).

4. Check on BP and pulse every 15 minutes, and record results carefully.

5. If he has a Foley, be sure it has a urometer; check urine output every 15-30 minutes. No Foley? Ask for an order, stat!

6. Keep a close eye on his monitor. This is open season for arrhythmias.

7. Bring the defibrillator near the bed. Screen it.

Exercise 35

What orders do you anticipate from Dr. Hart? In other words, what are you preparing for? List as many things as you can. (Answers follow this exercise).

1.

2.

3.

4.

5.

6.

Answers

1. Adjust IV flow rate according to his orders.

2. Insert Foley catheter if the patient doesn't have one.

3. Assist in drawing arterial blood gases, stat, and probably repeatedly.

4. Dr. Hart is on his way in. Get any lab, x-ray, and ECG findings assembled. Have the vital sign flow sheet ready for comparison.

5. You may need any of the drugs we discussed earlier.

6. What if Dr. Hart orders CVP or Swan-Ganz insertion? Do you know where the equipment is? If you don't know how to assist with insertion and calibration, do you know whom to call for help?

Exercise 36

Now Dr. Hart has done everything he can, short of inserting an IABP. It's "wait-and-see" time. He goes back to his office and you go back to the bedside. What will you be doing now? Well, let's see:

1. Keep a supercareful measurement of _____ and _____ to determine his fluid balance. — intake, output

2. Promptly and accurately administer all drugs, watching for _____ _____ . — side effects

3. Make repeated checks on vital signs and hemodynamic status; these may include _____, _____, _____, _____, _____, _____, and _____. — BP, P, CVP, UO, ABP, PAP, PCWP

4. You must keep all those IV lines _____ and adjust the drip to the right rate. — open

5. Keep a watchful eye on the monitor for _____ . — arrhythmias

6. Keep track of lab studies, especially _____ _____ _____ . — arterial blood gases

7. If respirations falter and hypoxia increases, you must anticipate insertion of an _____ _____ and _____ _____ . — endotracheal tube, assisted ventilation

8. You will need to _____ the patient's position hourly—not grossly, just tilting with pillows, but don't let him just lie there. — change

9. _____ with him. Don't you think he knows he's dying, or is very close to it? — Stay

After studying this moribund complication, do you feel the way I do? Sort of down-in-the-dumps? Maybe a walk in the fresh air or washing the dinner dishes (ugh!) will revive us. Then let's tackle the next complication of MI.

THROMBOEMBOLISM (*ICC, 4th ed., p. 110*)

Before we begin our discussion of thromboembolism, we must clarify a basic point. A *thrombus* is a clot sitting around the home fires. When a thrombus turns tramp, it becomes an embolus. An *embolus* roams through the circulatory system "just a-lookin' for a home."

If you're still confused, here's one more hint. You've seen the term *thromboembolism*, but have you ever seen *embothrombolism*? No, the thrombus comes first; it becomes an embolus only when it moves.

Exercise 37

1. After an MI, there seems to be an increased incidence of clots, or _____ .

thrombi

2. The thrombi forming in the deep veins of the legs are called _____ thrombi.

peripheral

3. Thrombi forming inside the heart's chambers are called _____ thrombi.

mural

4. Inactivity causing _____ _____ may lead to peripheral thrombus formation.

venous stasis

5. Coronary heart disease itself may be associated with an (increase/decrease) in clotting tendency.

increase

6. When a thrombus breaks loose and migrates, it's called an _____ .

embolus

7. Three sites where emboli may lodge are: _____ , _____ , _____ _____ .

lungs, brain
peripheral vessels

8. They're classified as _____ , _____ , or _____ emboli.

pulmonary, cerebral,
peripheral

PULMONARY EMBOLISM (*ICC, 4th ed., pp. 110-111*)

First, let's discuss emboli that lodge in the lungs. A large clot blocking off a major artery in the lungs produces unforgettable symptoms. Your patient is suddenly frantic for breath, shocky, apprehensive, and in terrible pain. Not all pulmonary emboli block off major arteries, so sometimes the picture is less grim.

I'd like to let a nurse friend of mine, Joan, tell what it's like to have a pulmonary emboli. Although her embolism wasn't caused by MI, the symptoms were the same. Joan says, "I'd just had a complete physical, and as I trotted out of the doctor's office, I was stabbed with a knifelike pain in my right chest, I know exactly what a patient means when he says, "the pain took my breath away.' But I didn't dare return to the doctor's office; I could just see the 'hypochondriac' label floating there." So Joan rationalized, "Must have pulled a muscle opening that door." By breathing "no deeper than the second intercostal space" she managed to get home to her heating pad.

The pain subsided, and the next day Joan and another nurse went to San Francisco to a California Nurses' Association council meeting—a good place for a second, less severe attack. The third attack came on the Golden Gate bridge in rush-hour traffic. Joan says, "I'd have gone to any hospital anywhere if we could have gotten off that bridge." But the pain subsided before the traffic jam did, and she made it home. "Go to the Emergency Room at midnight for a pain I'd had for 35 hours? No way!" So Joan went to bed with her faithful heating pad, only to awaken at 5 AM. "The knife again—the worst yet—so bad I couldn't sit up or reach the phone." She was drenched with perspiration and spitting up rusty, bloody sputum.

Joan's story ends with 16 days in the hospital, 6 weeks convalescence, and 6 months on anticoagulants.

Exercise 38

1. Most pulmonary emboli usually originate in the veins of the _____ .

legs

2. Trace their route: They start in the legs, go to the _____ vena cava, right _____ , right _____ , and finally to the _____ artery.

inferior
atrium, ventricle,
pulmonary

85

3. The clot doesn't pass through the lungs to the left atrium because _____ _____ .

pulmonary arteries are too small

4. If a small pulmonary artery branch is obstructed, there may be _____ symptoms.

no or minor

5. Obstruction of a main pulmonary artery usually causes _____ .

death

6. Pain from a pulmonary embolism usually (does/does not) radiate into the arms.

does not

7. The pain usually (is/is not) increased by deep inspiration.

is

8. In nearly all patients, the respiratory rate_____ and the heart rate _____ .

increases increases

9. With a stethoscope, you may hear _____ .

wheezing or rales

10. You will need to order a _____ _____ and _____ _____ _____ .

12-lead ECG, arterial blood gases

11. Radioactive_____ _____ is the best means of detecting a pulmonary embolism.

lung scanning

12. Mural thrombi form in the (left/right) ventricle after acute MI.

left

13. Mural thrombi (are/are not) likely to cause pulmonary embolism.

are not

CEREBRAL AND PERIPHERAL EMBOLISM
(*ICC, 4th ed., pp. 111-113*)

If, after an MI, an embolus finds a home in the cerebral arteries, what would you expect to happen? The picture of a stroke, right? (Can you think of anything worse than having an MI and a stroke together?) If a mural thrombus avoids a cerebral hang-up, it may swim through the systemic arteries until it finds one too small for navigation. This may be in the arms or legs or abdomen—in fact, anywhere in the arterial system.

Exercise 39

1. Clots originating in the left ventricle are called _____ thrombi.

mural

2. Mural thrombi travel from the left_____ through the_____ to the _____ or _____ arteries.

ventricle, aorta
cerebral, peripheral

3. A cerebral embolus may cause the picture of a _____ .

stroke

4. Acute MI and a cerebral embolism = a _____ prognosis.

poor

5. Why should an ECG be taken on patients admitted with a diagnosis of CVA?
_____
_____
_____
_____
_____ .

Because the CVA may be due to an embolism after MI. With aphasia they couldn't describe the chest pain, etc., that preceded the stroke.

6. Peripheral emboli most often lodge in the _____ or _____ arteries.

femoral, iliac

7. Signs of a peripheral embolus are a _____ , _____ , _____ extremity.

cold, pale, pulseless

8. If this occurs, you should promptly _____ _____ _____ .

notify the doctor

9. Immediate _____ may save the limb.

surgery

10. Again, the best treatment of any kind of embolism is_____ .

prevention

Exercise 40: Thromboembolism and Treatment

1. Venous stasis probably (increases/decreases) the chances of thrombus formation.

   increases

2. List 2 ways you can minimize venous stasis: _____ _____ , _____ .

   turn patient periodically, regular passive leg and arm exercises

3. Elastic _____ are used to prevent _____ _____ ; check them for smooth fit.

   stockings, venous pooling

4. Elevating the gatch or placing pillows under the knees (is/is not) advisable.

   is not

5. Drugs used to decrease clot formation are called _____ .

   anticoagulants

6. An overdose of anticoagulants may cause _____ .

   bleeding

7. Watch the patient closely for bleeding in_____ ,_____ , or_____ .

   skin, urine, stools

8. Heparin is usually given in a constant _____ drip.

   intravenous

9. Heparin is used to treat the embolus. (True/False)

   False

10. Heparin is used to _____ _____ of the embolus.

    prevent extension

11. A continuous heparin drip usually contains _____ units of heparin in 500 cc D$_5$W.

    20,000

12. The lab work ordered to check on clotting time will probably be an APTT, that is, _____ _____ _____ time.

    activated partial thromboplastic

13. Your patient's APTT should be _____ to _____ the normal control value.

    2, 2.5

14. You'd expect the doctor to order an APTT _____ to _____ hours after starting heparin and then _____ .

    4, 6
    daily

15. If you're using a heparin lock rather than a drip, the usual dosage is _____ to _____ units every _____ to _____ hours.

    5000
    10,000, 4, 6

16. Heparin dosage is adjusted by the doctor in accordance with the patient's_____ _____ .

    clotting
    time

17. The antidote (antagonist) for an overdose of heparin is _____ _____ , or Vitamin _____ .

    protamine
    sulfate, K$_1$

VENTRICULAR RUPTURE (*ICC, 4th ed., pp. 113-114*)

Exercise 41

1. The rupture may take place in the _____ wall (or free wall) of the ventricle.

   outer

2. Or it may occur in the _____ between the ventricles.

   septum

3. Ventricular rupture is usually associated with extensive_____ infarction.

   transmural

4. An outer wall rupture allows blood to leave the heart and fill the _____ _____ .

   pericardial
   sac

5. This rupture, which compresses or constricts the heart, is called _____ _____ .

   cardiac
   tamponade

6. This situation usually results in _____ .

   death

7. Even with a septal rupture, the prognosis is _____ _____ .

   very poor

8. Signs of septal rupture may include _____ _____ _____ and the development of a loud precordial _____ murmur.

   right heart failure
   systolic

9. If the patient survives, _____ _____ of the septal defect is possible.

10. The diagnosis of septal rupture can be confirmed by inserting a_____-_____ _____ .

CARDIAC ARRHYTHMIAS (*ICC, 4th ed., p. 114*)

We've saved the most common complication—arrhythmias—for last. In fact, all of the remaining chapters in *ICC,* 4th ed., are concerned with these disturbances of the electrical activity of the heart.

Once you've finished the crossword puzzle, word rounds, and definagram in this chapter, we'll begin our study of arrhythmias.

REVIEW (*ICC, 4th ed., Chapter 7*)

Exercise 42

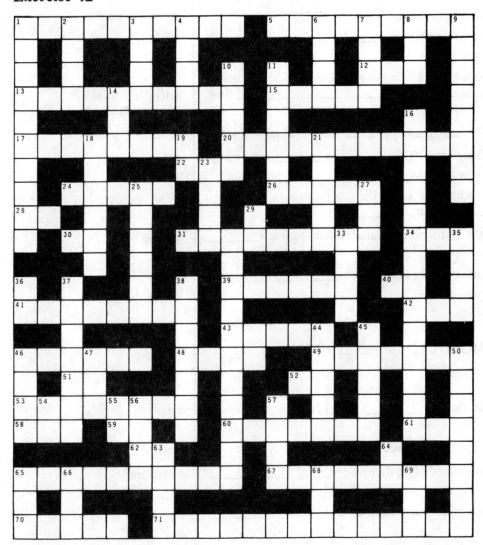

Figure 7.4. Crossword Puzzle.

ACROSS

1. Adjective describing a sudden attack: _____ .

5. Trade name for Ianatoside C-digitalis preparation: _____ .

12. _____ patients with massive pulmonary embolism survive.

88

13. Fast-acting diuretic: _____ acid.   ethacrynic

15. Not hidden, observable: _____ .   overt

17. Decreased urinary output: _____ .   oliguria

20. Rotating_____ can be used to treat acute pulmonary edema.   tourniquets

22. Most cardiogenic shock patients _____ .   die

24. Sudden acute right heart failure may be caused by_____ going through a septal rupture.   blood

26. CCU nurse will probably be the first to detect _____ heart failure.   early

28. Low-sodium diet = 1000 _____ sodium/day.   mg

30. Would you hear rales from interstitial edema? _____   no

31. The plural of embolus is emboli, not _____ .   embolisms

34. Pulmonary (abbreviation): _____ .   pul

39. With acute pulmonary edema the patient _____ incessantly.   coughs

40. Registered nurse (abbreviation): _____ .   RN

41. Paroxysmal nocturnal dyspnea starts _____ .   suddenly

42. With PND most patients want to _____ in bed.   sit

43. Pedal edema may be a symptom of _____ heart failure.   right

46. End product of anaerobic metabolism: _____ acid.   lactic

48. A CCU nurse keeps careful _____ on her patients (slang).   tabs

49. Right upper quadrant abdominal pain may mean _____ engorgement during right heart failure.   hepatic

51. Prefix meaning to restore to a previous condition: _____ .   re

52. Ultimate treatment for ventricular rupture takes place in_____ (abbreviation).   OR

53. Pertaining to course of disease or to symptoms: _____ .   clinical

58. Only nearest _____ are usually allowed to visit in CCU.   kin

59. Are hypotension and cardiogenic shock the same? _____ .   no

60. Normal cellular metabolism using oxygen: _____ .   aerobic

61. Prevention and treatment of complications is the _____ (slang) of CCU.   nub

62. Orally (abbreviation): _____ .   PO

65. Generic name for Lasix: _____ .   furosemide

67. Symptoms of cardiogenic shock result from decreased tissue _____.   perfusion

70. Right heart failure symptoms are related to retention of sodium and _____ .   water

71. Adjective pertaining to blocking of blood vessels by an embolus: _____.   thromboembolic

DOWN

1. Venesection, withdrawing blood: _____.   phlebotomy

2. Compassion, pity—used with suffixes "less" or "full" (latter-archaic):_____ .   ruth-

3. It is _____ responsibility to detect early complications in an MI patient.   your

4. Be sure the anxious patient understands what you_____ by your explanations.   mean

6. Very little can be _____ to reverse cardiogenic shock.   done

7. The _____ ventricle is most often affected by an MI.   left

8. The _____ concept in CCU is prevention.   new

9. Increased urinary output: _____ .   diuresis

10. At the point of decompensation, _____ heart failure occurs.   acute

11. Stroke _____ × heart rate = cardiac output.   volume

14. System responsible for reducing MI death rate: _____ .   CCU

16. Failure to make up for a defect: _____ .   decompensation

18. Third heart sound associated with left ventricular failure: _____ .   gallop

19. Prefix meaning "to" or "toward": _____ .   ad

21. What a CCU nurse smells trouble with: _____ . (Latin)   nares

23. The nurse is the most important _____ in a good CCU.   item

25. Is helpful in treating PND: _____ .   oxygen

27. Do MI patients die from complications? _____   yes

29. Is bradycardia an early sign of heart failure? _____   no

32. Sodium _____ is used to control acidosis.   bicarbonate

33. Face covering worn in surgery: _____ .   mask

35. _____ ventricular failure usually comes first.   Left

36. Abbreviation for sulfate of an opium alkaloid: _____ .   ms

37. Powerful diuretic (brand name): _____ .   Edecrin

38. Contraction phase of cardiac cycle: _____ .   systole

44. To beat rapidly, rhythmically; to pound: _____ .   throb

45. Most vital nerve if nurse is to see the "faces of fear": _____ .   optic

46. _____ of potassium predisposes to ventricular arrhythmias.   Lack

47. Only about _____% of MI patients will have no arrhythmias.   10

50. End product of aerobic metabolism: _____ acid.   carbonic

54. Symbol for lithium: _____ .   LI

55. Type of drugs that strengthen myocardial contraction (first two letters): _____ .   in

56. The patient may use denial to _____ with fears.   cope

57. Rotating tourniquets are used to _____ blood in the extremities.   trap

63. Don't _____ skin inspection on the patient receiving anticoagulants.   omit

64. Abbreviation for hour of sleep: _____ .   hs

65. _____ patients with ventricular rupture survive.   Few

66. What CCU nurses must avoid in their thinking: _____ .   rut

68. MI patients may _____ the fact that they haven't controlled the risk factors.   rue

69. Patient with acute heart failure is very _____ .   ill

90

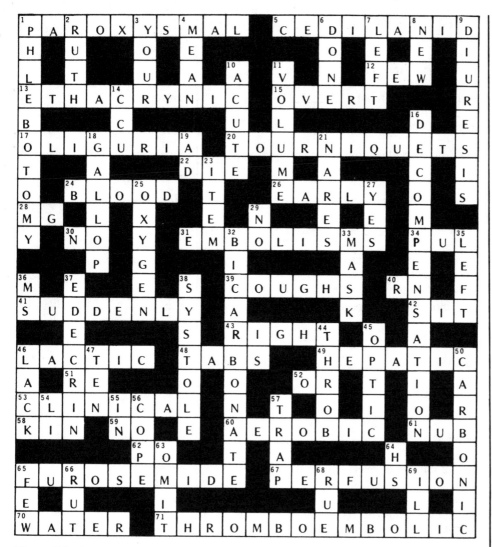

Figure 7.5. Answers.

Exercise 43

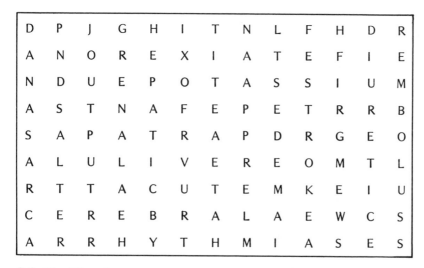

Figure 7.6. Word Rounds.

Complete the statements below, then locate your answer in the scrambled letters. Words are spelled from left to right, or downward.

1. _____ and nausea may be caused by hepatic engorgement.   Anorexia

91

2. Left ventricular failure that often develops abruptly during sleep (abbreviation): ________ .

PND

3. Retention of water and ________ characterizes right heart failure.

salt

4. Generalized edema found in severe right heart failure: ______________ .

anasarca

5. Cardiac ______________ is markedly reduced in cardiogenic shock.

output

6. Decreased ______________ blood flow and kidney function characterize cardiogenic shock.

renal

7. ______________ engorgement may occur with severe right heart failure.

Hepatic

8. Usually restricted in CCU diets (symbol): ________ .

Na

9. ______________________ depletion from diuretics may cause ventricular arrhythmias.

Potassium

10. Rotating tourniquets can ________ blood in the extremities.

trap

11. May be engorged in severe right heart failure: ______________ .

liver

12. When decompensation is reached, the patient is in ______________ heart failure.

acute

13. Inadequate ______________ perfusion causes some of the early symptoms of cardiogenic shock.

cerebral

14. Most frequent complication after an MI: ______________________ .

arrhythmias

15. Alveolar ______________ is a sign of clinical or overt left ventricular failure.

edema

16. Mural thrombi reaching the brain may cause ______________ symptoms.

stroke

17. Drug used to increase urinary output: ______________ .

diuretic

18. A large pulmonary ______________ may cause severe symptoms and death.

embolus

19. Swan-Ganz pressure reading taken with the balloon inflated (abbreviation): ______________ .

PCWP

20. Swan-Ganz pressure reading taken with the balloon deflated (abbreviation): ________ .

PAP

D	P	J	G	H	I	T	N	L	F	H	D	R
A	N	O	R	E	X	I	A	T	E	F	I	E
N	D	U	E	P	O	T	A	S	S	I	U	M
A	S	T	N	A	F	E	P	E	T	R	R	B
S	A	P	A	T	R	A	P	D	R	G	E	O
A	L	U	L	I	V	E	R	E	O	M	T	L
R	T	T	A	C	U	T	E	M	K	E	I	U
C	E	R	E	B	R	A	L	A	E	W	C	S
A	R	R	H	Y	T	H	M	I	A	S	E	S

Figure 7.7. Answers.

Exercise 45

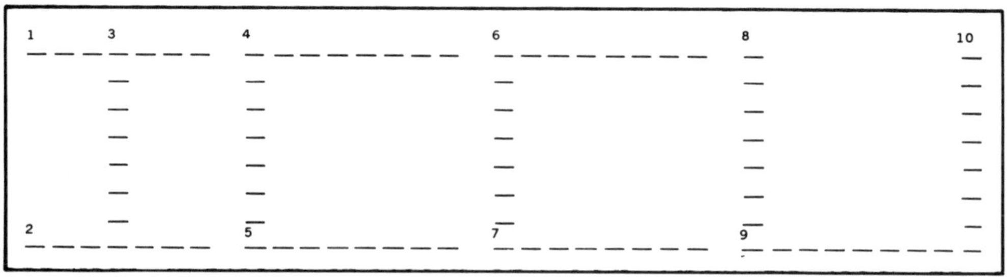

Figure 7.8. Definagram.

Complete the following definitions. Place your answers beside the corresponding number in the definagram.

ACROSS

1. Abnormal particles migrating through the bloodstream. _____.   embolus

2. Inability to express oneself through speech: _____ .   aphasia

4. Lack of oxygen in the blood: _____ .   anoxemia

5. Generalized edema of the body: _____ .   anasarca

6. Pertaining to the air sacs of the lungs: _____ .   alveolar

7. Pertaining to the contraction phase of cardiac cycle: _____ .   systolic

9. Without free oxygen: _____ .   anaerobic

DOWN

3. Diminished amount and frequency of urine: _____.   oliguria

4. Loss of appetite: _____ .   anorexia

6. Can be caused by retention of lactic acid: _____ .   acidosis

8. Insufficient oxygenation of an area: _____ .   ischemia

10. Acid end product of an aerobic metabolism: _____ .   carbonic

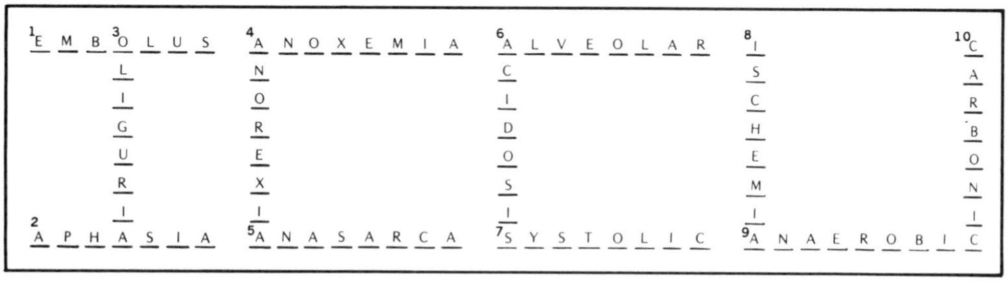

Figure 7.9. Answers.

93

8

The
Electrocardiographic
Interpretation of
Arrhythmias

FUNDAMENTALS OF
ELECTROCARDIOGRAPHY
(ICC, 4th ed., pp. 115-116)

Welcome to the fascinating world of monitoring! Before long, I hope monitors will become your best friend. Perhaps you've wondered why such a fuss is made over the diagnosis of arrhythmias. Simply, because arrhythmias can kill.

And why do we worry about the *type* or classification of arrhythmias we're seeing? Because different arrhythmias require different treatments. Some are dangerous; some are not dangerous. And some arrhythmias require no treatment.

Before we begin, please, let me convince you of one thing. You can't just memorize arrhythmia patterns from this or any other book. You can't look at p. 123, figure 8.10 in *ICC*, 4th ed., for example, and say, "That's the way all normal sinus rhythms (NSR) will look. Anything else is an arrhythmia and should be treated." None of your patients looks exactly alike physically—why should they be identical electrically?

You must take time to learn the meaning of each part of the electrical patterns and know the limits of normal. Then be familiar with the diagnostic criteria for each arrhythmia; but, please, don't try to just memorize patterns. I know of no shortcuts to interpreting arrhythmias. One thing is certain: You must be able to recognize *normal* before you can diagnose *abnormal*.

We'll go through this important chapter step by step, using a series of questions and answers.

Exercise 1

Label Figure 8.1 showing the electrical system of the heart.

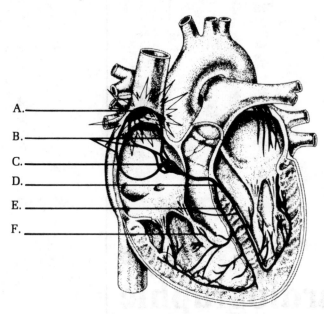

A._____

B._____

C._____

D._____

E._____

F._____

A. SA node

B. Internodal tracts

C. AV node

D. Bundle of His

E. Right and left bundle branches

F. Purkinje fibers

Figure 8.1.

How did you do? If you made any mistakes, stop here and reread the material in *ICC*, 4th ed. You won't be able to understand arrhythmias unless you are absolutely sure about the conduction pathway.

Exercise 2

1. The normal pacemaker of the heart is in the _____ node.

   sinoatrial (SA)

2. The SA node normally discharges an electrical force_____ to_____ times per minute.

   60, 100

3. Right now (if you're normal), your heart rate is being controlled by the_____.

   SA node

4. Your heart rate is probably between_____ and_____.

   60, 100

5. The electrical impulse leaves the SA node and travels through the _____ _____, ____ _____, _____ ____ _____, _____ _____, and _____ _____, and finally stimulates the cells at the Purkinje-myocardial junction to discharge their stored electrical forces, causing a ventricular contraction.

   internodal tracts, AV node, Bundle of His, bundle branches, Purkinje fibers

6. The discharge of electrical forces causing this contraction is called
   _____.

   depolarization

7. After depolarization, the rest or recovery period is called _____. (If you have trouble with this, associate the *re* in *re*polarization with *re*st or *re*covery.)

   repolarization

8. The pacemaking function of the SA node can be taken over by an _____ pacemaker.

   ectopic

9. The various phases of the cardiac cycle can be identified on an _____.

   ECG

10. The electrocardiogram records the _____ forces from the heart that are transmitted to the body's surface.

    electrical

11. Identify which is the machine and which is the printed record.
    A. Electrocardiogram: _____

    record

    B. Electrocardiograph: _____
       (Just remember tele*graph*/tele*gram*. Now, if you've got that, let's use ECG for both machine and record—it's so much easier!)

    machine

LIMB LEADS AND MONITORING LEADS
(ICC, 4th ed., pp. 117-118)

I'm sure you've watched technicians taking an ECG, and you know that they strap little electrodes on all 4 limbs. Then they place another electrode on the chest wall and move it from place to place. The purpose of these multiple electrodes is to get several different views of the heart's electrical activity. In fact, by simply switching a knob on the ECG machine, 12 separate views—or leads—can be obtained. This is called a 12-lead electrocardiogram. Each lead shows a different electrical pattern on the ECG, as the flow of current being recorded is from different electrode positions.

We'll discuss only the 3 leads called the *standard limb leads* because they are recorded from the limb electrodes. Actually, only 3 of the 4 limb electrodes are "working" electrodes. The fourth, on the right leg, is only a ground wire, so we can ignore it. Now if we take the 3 working electrodes—those on the right arm, left arm, and left leg—and join them in a theoretical triangle, we can see the 3 limb leads (Figure 8.2). I could never really picture this until I wrote the numerals I, II, and III on 6 pieces of tape and put them on my shoulders and left thigh. Then I could "see" Einthoven's triangle. If you're confused, try it. Then complete the following exercise.

Exercise 3

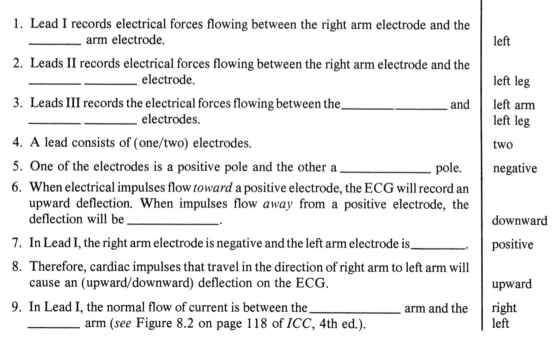

Figure 8.2. Einthoven's triangle.

1. Lead I records electrical forces flowing between the right arm electrode and the _____ arm electrode.

   left

2. Leads II records electrical forces flowing between the right arm electrode and the _____ _____ electrode.

   left leg

3. Leads III records the electrical forces flowing between the_____ _____ and _____ _____ electrodes.

   left arm
   left leg

4. A lead consists of (one/two) electrodes.

   two

5. One of the electrodes is a positive pole and the other a _____ pole.

   negative

6. When electrical impulses flow *toward* a positive electrode, the ECG will record an upward deflection. When impulses flow *away* from a positive electrode, the deflection will be _____.

   downward

7. In Lead I, the right arm electrode is negative and the left arm electrode is_____.

   positive

8. Therefore, cardiac impulses that travel in the direction of right arm to left arm will cause an (upward/downward) deflection on the ECG.

   upward

9. In Lead I, the normal flow of current is between the _____ arm and the _____ arm (*see* Figure 8.2 on page 118 of *ICC*, 4th ed.).

   right
   left

97

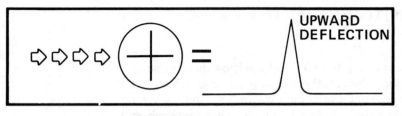

CURRENT FLOW   ELECTRODES

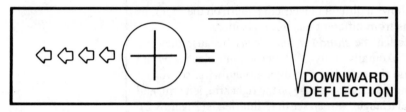

Figure 8.3. Current flowing *toward* a positive electrode causes a positive inflection. Current flowing *away* from a positive electrode causes a negative deflection.

10. Normally, Lead I should cause an _____ deflection on the ECG.   upward

11. In Lead II, the right arm electrode is negative and the left electrode is _____.   positive

12. Cardiac impulses flowing from the right arm toward the left leg will cause an _____ deflection on the ECG.   upward

13. This represents the normal flow of current in Lead II. However, if for some reason impulses flowed *away* from the left leg (the positive electrode), the deflection would be _____.   downward

14. In Lead III, either the left arm or left leg can be the positive electrode, depending on the position (or axis) of the heart. If the left leg electrode is positive, the right arm will then be _____.   negative

15. In this case, impulses from the heart traveling in the direction of left arm to left leg will cause an _____ deflection on the ECG.   upward

16. But if impulses travel in the opposite direction (from left leg to left arm), the deflection will be _____.   downward

Remember: current flowing *toward* a positive electrode causes an upward (or positive) deflection and impulses flowing *away* from a positive electrode cause a downward (or negative) deflection.

All of this brings us to cardiac monitoring. Monitors use just one lead for detecting arrhythmias. The lead is determined by where you place the electrodes on your patient's chest. Although the electrodes are on the chest rather than the limbs, the principles we just discussed still hold true.

CARDIAC CYCLE TERMS (*ICC, 4th ed., p. 118*)

In Figure 8.3 you'll see a graph with a series of little bumps, bigger bumps, and tall, narrow spikes.

Before I took my CCU course, I had patients on monitors, but I had no idea of what I was seeing or even any idea of how to describe it. One day, the ECG pattern suddenly looked very different, and in panic I called the doctor and said, "You'd better come quick, there are too many little squiggles and not enough big wiggles."

Obviously, we need names for those bumps. And if you've ever tired of diagrams labeled a, b, c—take heart; for these deflections we use letters that make even less sense!

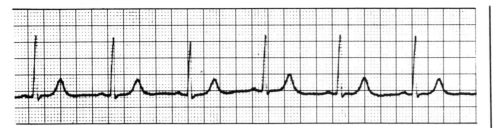

Figure 8.4.

Exercise 4

1. The cardiac cycle involves two phases: _____ and
   _____.

   depolarization
   repolarization

2. The ECG records the _____ _____ during the
   cardiac cycle.

   electrical activity

3. The electrical activity creates a series of deflections (waves) on the ECG that are
   labeled _____, _____, _____, _____, and _____.

   P, Q, R, S, T

4. The ECG allows us to measure the _____ of these
   waves.

   amplitude or voltage

5. It also allows us to measure the _____ of the waves.

   duration

ECG MEASUREMENTS (*ICC, 4th ed., pp. 118-119*)

ECGs are recorded on graph paper that moves through the machine at a constant
speed. Without this standardized graph paper, it would be difficult to measure either the
amplitude or the duration of the various waves. The graph simplifies things—if you can
graph temperatures, you'll be able to understand ECG measurements. So suppose we
take some temps at 8 AM, 12 noon, 4 PM, and 8 PM, and graph them. Now compare this
graph with an ECG.

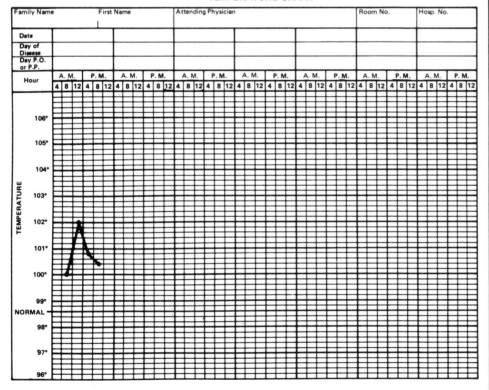

Figure 8.5. Temperature graph.

99

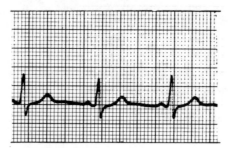

Figure 8.6. ECG.

Exercise 5

1. Your temp graph tells you and the doctor two things: the _____ you took the temperature and the _____ of temperature.

   time

   degree or amount

2. The ECG graph also tells two things: the _____ (or duration) of an electrical impulse and the _____ of its voltage.

   time

   amount

3. Time lines on your temp graph run up and down, or _____.

   vertically

4. Similarly, time lines on the ECG run up and down, or _____.

   vertically

5. This means that the distance from one vertical line to the next vertical line on a temp graph or an ECG measures an interval of _____.

   time

6. Amount of temperature is read on lines running across, or _____ on the graph.

   horizontally

7. Amount of voltage is shown on an ECG by lines running across, or

   _____.

   horizontally

8. Thus, an ECG allows the amplitude, or_____, of an electrical wave to be measured.

   voltage

9. It also shows how much_____ it took for an impulse to travel through the heart.

   time

Exercise 6

1. If your patient's temperature goes up, the graph line goes _____.

   up

2. On an ECG, an increase in voltage is shown by a line going_____.

   up

3. On a temp graph, temperature is measured in units called _____.

   degrees

4. On an ECG, voltage is measured in units called _____.

   millivolts

5. One small square on an ECG graph (the space between two horizontal lines) equals _____ millimeter (mm).

   1

6. One millimeter represents one-tenth of a _____.

   millivolt

7. How many squares high is the deflection in Figure 8.7? _____.

   10

8. This equals _____ millimeters.

   10

9. Or how many millivolts? _____

   1 millivolt $(10 \times 0.1 = 1)$

10. In order to save your eyesight (and sanity), you can remember that there are _____ little squares enclosed in a darker line or a big square.

    5

11. Thus, two large squares equal _____ millimeters, or _____ millivolt.

    10, 1

12. The voltage of the deflection in Figure 8.8 is _____ millivolts.

    1.4 millivolts $(14 \times 0.1 = 1.4)$

13. The voltage of the deflection in Figure 8.9 is _____ millivolts.

    0.6 millivolts $(6 \times 0.1 = 0.6)$

100

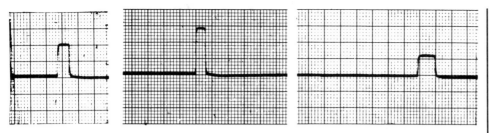

Figure 8.7.   **Figure 8.8.**   **Figure 8.9.**

Exercise 7

You're doing fine. Now let's leave voltage and go on to time.

1. On the temp graph, time is shown in intervals of _____.

    hours

2. On an ECG, time is shown in intervals of _____ of a _____. (Wow! Think about that.)

    hundredths, second

3. One small square (the space between 2 vertical lines) equals _____ seconds.

    0.04 (four hundredths)

4. Four small squares = _____ seconds.

    0.16

5. Five small squares = _____ seconds.

    0.20

6. 0.20 seconds is the same as _____ tenths of a second. (If you're weak on decimals, better review them until you're sure the above makes sense.)

    two

7. How many small squares are enclosed in darker lines to form a larger square? _____.

    5

8. Five small squares = _____ seconds.

    0.20

9. One large square = _____ seconds.

    0.20

10. What is the duration of the deflection in Figure 8.10? _____

    0.24 seconds
    (6 small boxes × 0.04 seconds)

11. What is the duration of the actual wave in Figure 8.11? _____

    0.04 seconds
    (1 small box × 0.04 seconds)

12. What about the wave in Figure 8.12? (Don't let it fool you just because it's a downward (negative) wave. You count the time the same way.) _____

    0.16 seconds
    (4 small boxes × 0.04 seconds)

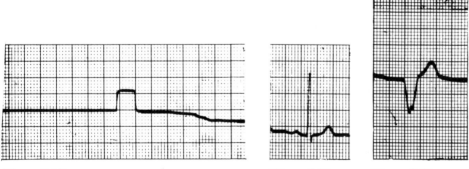

Figure 8.10.   **Figure 8.11.**   **Figure 8.12.**

ECG MEASUREMENT PRACTICE
(*ICC, 4th ed., pp. 118-119*)

If you've plodded through this far on your own, I think you're simply marvelous. Now we can proceed to put this information to practical use.

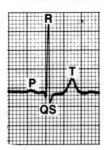

Figure 8.13. Use this ECG in answering the questions in Exercise 8.

Exercise 8

1. What is the duration of the P wave? _____   about 2 small boxes or 0.08 seconds

2. What is the duration of the QRS complex? _____   1 small box or 0.04 seconds

3. What is the duration of the T wave? _____   about 4 small boxes or 0.16 seconds

4. What is the duration of the entire cardiac cycle (from the beginning of the P wave to the end of the T wave)? _____   14 small boxes or 0.56 seconds

5. What is the voltage of the P wave? _____   less than 1 small box or less than 0.1 millivolt

6. What is the voltage of the R wave? _____   18 small boxes or 1.8 millivolts

7. Which waves have positive deflections? _____   P, R, and T

8. Which waves have negative deflections? _____   Q and S

CARDIAC CYCLE ON THE ECG
(ICC, 4th ed., pp. 120-124)

Now we'll analyze each of the separate waves and segments of the ECG to see what they represent.

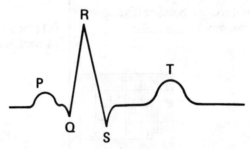

Figure 8.14. Normal cardiac cycle. (Refer to this figure in Exercises 9–12.)

Exercise 9

1. A normal P wave tells you that the electrical impulse started in the _____ node.   SA

2. So, with a normal sinus pacemaker, you'd see a normal _____ wave on the ECG.   P

3. "Normal" means normal in _____ and _____.   size, shape

4. If a P wave is not present, it means the pacemaker (is/is not) in the SA node.   is not

5. Aberrantly shaped P waves mean that the configuration of the waves is _____.   abnormal or distorted

6. Aberrant P waves may indicate that the pacemaker (is/is not) in the SA node.   is not

102

You should realize that there is a wide range for normal. Just because a P wave, or any other wave, doesn't look just like the picture in a textbook, you can't say that something is wrong. Each patient's "normal" is as unique as fingerprints. You'll soon develop a feel for the range of normal.

Exercise 10

We need to know something about the period from the beginning of the P wave to the beginning of the QRS complex, that is, the PR interval. Try these:

1. The PR interval is measured from the _____ of the P wave to the _____ of the QRS complex. (Just like timing a labor contraction—from the beginning of one to the beginning of the next).

   beginning
   beginning

2. The PR interval represents the passage of the electrical impulse from the _____ node through the _____ through the _____ node to the ventricles.

   SA
   atrium, AV

3. The normal PR should be between _____ to _____ seconds. (Memorize the normal time limits. Though some doctors and books may use slightly different figures, 0.10 to 0.20 are easy to learn and you can modify them later if you need to.)

   0.10, 0.20

4. A delay in the impulse passing the AV node might make the PR (more/less) than 0.20 seconds.

   more

5. Calculate the PR interval in Figure 8.15. _____

   0.16 seconds

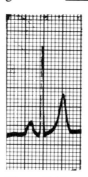

Figure 8.15.

Note: If the complex (cardiac cycle) you're interpreting has a Q wave (the downward deflection), you calculate the PR to the beginning of the Q wave. If there is no Q wave, calculate to the R wave. The Q wave is absent in some leads and hard to see in others, so don't worry about it.

Exercise 11

1. The QRS complex represents the depolarization of the _____.

   ventricles

2. The large positive deflection is the _____ wave.

   R

3. If there is a negative deflection before the R wave, it's called a _____ wave.

   Q

4. Sometimes the _____ wave may be absent.

   Q

5. The downward deflection after the R wave is called the _____ wave.

   S

6. The total QRS should not be longer than _____ seconds.

   0.12

7. In other words, it should take the electrical impulse no longer than _____ seconds to race through the ventricle.

   0.12

8. Ventricular depolarization should take less than _____ seconds.

   0.12

9. A QRS longer than 0.12 seconds indicates _____ conduction in the ventricles.

   abnormal or delayed

Exercise 12

1. Depolarization of the ventricles shows in the _____ complex.

   QRS

2. Repolarization of the ventricles shows in the _____ wave.

   T

3. Repolarization means: _____ recovery or rest period after contraction

4. The interval between the end of depolarization and the beginning of repolarization is called the _____ segment.   ST

5. The normal ST segment is (isoelectric/negative/positive). (Isoelectric means the dividing line between negative and positive. The deflection is neither upward nor downward but, rather, a straight line.)   isoelectric

6. An elevated (positive) or depressed (negative) ST may indicate muscle _____.   injury

7. An abnormal ST segment means that there is a delay in_____.   repolarization

8. One cause of this is _____ _____ _____.   acute myocardial infarction

9. The ST segment in Figure 8.16 is (depressed/elevated/isoelectric).   depressed

10. The T wave in Figure 8.17 is _____.   inverted

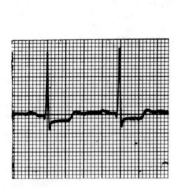

Figure 8.16.   **Figure 8.17.**

Exercise 13

1. The QT interval is measured from the _____ of the Q wave to the _____ of the T wave.   beginning / end

2. The QT shows the total time of _____ depolarization and repolarization.   ventricular

3. The QT duration (in normal sinus rhythm) seldom exceeds _____ seconds.   0.40

4. The QT in Figures 8.16 and 8.17 appears to be less than 0.40. (It's hard to see clearly.) This is (normal/abnormal).   normal

ECG INTERPRETATION (*ICC, 4th ed., pp. 120-124*)

Exercise 14

You've been working so hard, I think you deserve a treat. So let's visit a CCU. I want you to meet Nurse Dora Dom, who, poor dear, doesn't have a copy of this book. There are 5 patients on the monitors here, and I'll run a rhythm strip of each one for you. These are not textbook pictures, but real strips from actual patients.

Now, together, let's check all 5 patients. Join in the conversation and finish what "you" starts to say.

Figure 8.18.
Strip 1

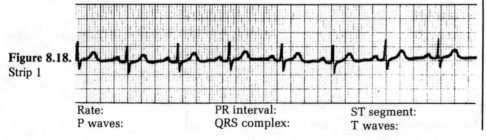

Rate: PR interval: ST segment:
P waves: QRS complex: T waves:

104

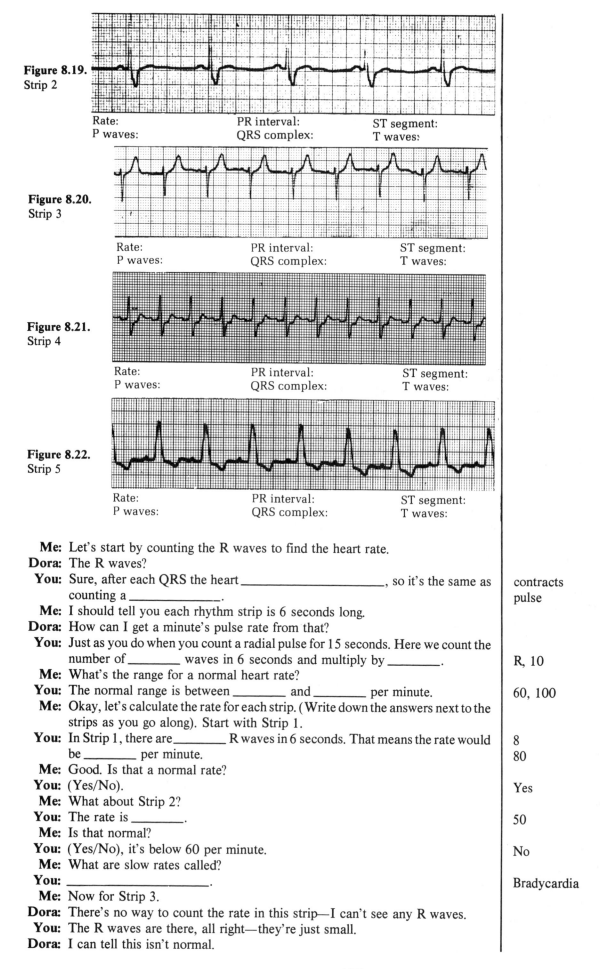

Figure 8.19.
Strip 2

Rate: PR interval: ST segment:
P waves: QRS complex: T waves:

Figure 8.20.
Strip 3

Rate: PR interval: ST segment:
P waves: QRS complex: T waves:

Figure 8.21.
Strip 4

Rate: PR interval: ST segment:
P waves: QRS complex: T waves:

Figure 8.22.
Strip 5

Rate: PR interval: ST segment:
P waves: QRS complex: T waves:

Me: Let's start by counting the R waves to find the heart rate.

Dora: The R waves?

You: Sure, after each QRS the heart _____, so it's the same as counting a _____.   contracts / pulse

Me: I should tell you each rhythm strip is 6 seconds long.

Dora: How can I get a minute's pulse rate from that?

You: Just as you do when you count a radial pulse for 15 seconds. Here we count the number of _____ waves in 6 seconds and multiply by _____.   R, 10

Me: What's the range for a normal heart rate?

You: The normal range is between _____ and _____ per minute.   60, 100

Me: Okay, let's calculate the rate for each strip. (Write down the answers next to the strips as you go along). Start with Strip 1.

You: In Strip 1, there are _____ R waves in 6 seconds. That means the rate would be _____ per minute.   8 / 80

Me: Good. Is that a normal rate?

You: (Yes/No).   Yes

Me: What about Strip 2?

You: The rate is _____.   50

Me: Is that normal?

You: (Yes/No), it's below 60 per minute.   No

Me: What are slow rates called?

You: _____.   Bradycardia

Me: Now for Strip 3.

Dora: There's no way to count the rate in this strip—I can't see any R waves.

You: The R waves are there, all right—they're just small.

Dora: I can tell this isn't normal.

105

Me: How do you know?	
Dora: It doesn't look like the pattern of normal in *ICC*, 4th ed. I know it by heart.	
Me: Not all normals look alike. You can't decide on that basis. You have to go step by step to see if anything is wrong.	
Dora: Well, something's wrong with the R wave.	
You: Maybe the R waves are small because of the position of the _____.	electrodes
Me: That's right. Remember what we said about how different leads give a different pattern? In this case, the R waves are small and the S waves are big because of the lead being used. Let's get back to the heart rate.	
You: It's _____ per minute.	90
Me: Normal or abnormal?	
You: _____.	Normal
Me: Strip 4 is very interesting. What's the rate here?	
You: It's _____ per minute.	120
Me: Normal?	
You: _____, it's greater than _____ per minute.	No, 100
Me: What are fast rates called?	
You: _____.	Tachycardia
Me: What's the rate in Strip 5?	
You: _____ per minute, which is _____.	80, normal
Me: Fine. You've learned a lot. Now let's analyze the P waves in each strip. Take a look at all of them and then write down whether they're normal or not.	
Dora: I don't like some of them. Strips 1 and 2 seem okay, but Strip 3 is very tiny. And the shapes of Strips 4 and 5 aren't smooth and rounded.	
Me: Who guaranteed that all P waves would be smooth and rounded or that they would have a certain "normal" height?	
You: I think P waves in Strips _____, _____, _____, _____, _____, are probably within normal limits.	1, 2, 3, 4, 5
Me: Again, the configuration of the wave depends a lot on the lead being recorded. Many times you can't be sure if it's normal from a single monitor lead.	
Dora: Does that mean we're through?	
Me: We've only discussed rate and P waves. Now measure the PR intervals and write down their duration.	
Dora: Where do you measure from? I forgot.	
You: The PR interval is measured from the _____ of the _____ wave to the beginning of the _____ complex.	beginning, P QRS
Me: What are the normal values?	
You: From _____ second to _____ second.	0.10, 0.20
Me: Are the PR intervals normal in these strips?	
You: _____.	Yes
Me: We're up to the QRS complex.	
Dora: How do we know if the QRS's are normal? They've got different shapes.	
You: You measure from the _____ of the complex to the _____ of the _____.	beginning end, S wave
Dora: Suppose there's no Q or S wave, then what do you do?	
You: You measure the _____.	R wave
Me: What is the normal duration of the QRS?	
You: It should be less than _____ seconds.	0.12
Me: Measure each QRS and write down your answers. Are they all normal?	
You: _____. In Strips _____ and _____ the QRS are _____.	No, 2, 5, prolonged
Me: What does that mean?	
You: There is some delay in _____ _____.	ventricular conduction
Me: Good thinking.	
Dora: I think you missed one. In Strip 3 the QRS is only one small box or 0.04 second, as far as I can see. So there's something wrong with that one, too.	
You: Nothing's wrong with the R wave, but you didn't include the _____ wave in your measurement.	S
Me: You have to measure the entire QRS complex.	

Dora: Does the QRS show depolarization or repolarization of the muscle? I never can remember the difference.

You: It means _____.

depolarization

Me: Now let's look at the ST segments.

Dora: I don't remember learning a time interval for the ST segment.

Me: You're right. We didn't learn one. We're interested in the position of the segment rather than its duration. It's very important.

You: I remember—the normal ST should not be negative or positive, it should be _____.

isoelectric

Me: Very good. If it's elevated or depressed, that's a sign of injury. What causes that?

You: One cause is _____ _____.

myocardial infarction

Me: So far, so good. Now, let's go over the ST segments. Lay a piece of paper across the baseline and see if the ST segment is above or below the baseline. In other words, is the segment elevated, depressed, or isoelectric? Write down your answers for each strip.

Dora: Strip 1 is okay.

Me: What did you write down about the others? Are they normal?

You: _____. The ST segments are_____ in Strips_____.

No, depressed, 4 and 5

Me: We're finally up to the T wave. Look at the T wave in the 5 strips.

Dora: They all look different. I don't understand that.

Me: There are many things that affect the T waves, and you can't expect them to look alike in each patient. We're interested mostly in whether the T waves are upright or inverted.

Dora: Why do we care about that?

You: Inverted T waves may be a sign of myocardial _____.

ischemia

Me: Right. But don't forget there are other causes as well. Now describe whether the T waves on the 5 strips are inverted or upright.

You: _____
_____.

They're inverted in Strip 5 and upright in all the others

Me: Were your answers right? Good. Let's celebrate! You've really got it!

Dora: *Celebrate*? Does that mean look at more ECGs?

THE IMPORTANCE OF THE ECG (*ICC, 4th ed., p. 124*)

Exercise 15

For variety's sake let's try some true and false questions. Complete *all* the questions before you check the answers.

1. People with normal ECGs can be assured that their immediate futures will be free from heart attacks.

False

2. Coronary atherosclerosis can be diagnosed early by ECG changes.

False

3. Ventricular systole (contraction) is shown on the ECG.

False

4. Myocardial ischemia can be recognized on the ECG.

True

5. The ECG shows only electrical activity.

True

6. The ECG clearly demonstrates the physical status of the heart.

False

7. The results of necrosis from previous MIs can be seen on an ECG.

True

8. Ventricular systole coincides with the peak of the QRS.

True

9. Ventricular diastole coincides with the end of the T to the next R.

True

10. The ECG shows both electrical and mechanical activity.

False

107

ARRHYTHMIAS: THEIR CLASSIFICATION
(ICC, 4th ed., pp. 125-126)

Exercise 16

1. Technically, the word *arrhythmia* means _____ of normal rhythm. — absence

2. In practice, however, we often mean any disturbance of _____, _____, or _____. — rate, rhythm, conduction

3. *ICC*, 4th ed., explains that arrhythmias are due to disturbances of _____ formation and disturbances of _____. — impulse conduction

4. Normally, impulses are initiated by the _____ _____. — SA node

5. Other sites where impulses can originate include the _____, _____ nodal area, and _____. — atria, AV ventricles

6. Thus, one way of classifying those arrhythmias caused by disturbances of impulse formation is by the _____ of origin. — site

7. Further classification of arrhythmias caused by disturbances of impulse formation is by the _____ of the disturbance. — mechanism

8. If the arrhythmia has an abnormally fast rate, it is called a _____. — tachycardia

9. If the arrhythmia has an abnormally slow rate, it is called a _____. — bradycardia

10. The mechanism can involve some impulses coming sooner than normal. These are called _____ beats. — premature

11. Two extremely rapid mechanisms of impulse formation are _____ and _____. These can originate either in the atria or in the ventricles. — flutter fibrillation

12. Classification of arrhythmias due to conduction disturbances refers to _____ _____ in the passage of the impulses. — blocks or delays

13. Conduction disturbance blocks can occur anywhere from the_____ node clear through to the _____. — SA ventricles

14. However, blocks are classified according to 3 main sites (from the top of the heart down):

    A. Blocks *within* the _____ node and _____. — SA, atria

    B. Blocks *between* the _____ and _____. — atria, ventricles

    C. Blocks *within* the _____. — ventricles

15. If we classify arrhythmias according to their seriousness, the most dangerous are labeled _____ arrhythmias. — lethal

16. The least serious arrhythmias are called _____ arrhythmias. — minor

17. In between these 2 groups is a third group of arrhythmias that are dangerous and require prompt treatment but are not immediately lethal. These are called_____ arrhythmias. — major

INTERPRETATION OF ARRHYTHMIAS
(ICC, 4th ed., pp. 127-131)

Exercise 17

Use the 5 steps listed here to interpret the following ECG. Don't worry about the actual diagnosis; you'll learn that later on. For now, be happy you understand the procedure involved in establishing a diagnosis. That's really progress.

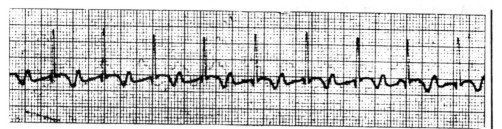

Figure 8.23.

STEP 1. CALCULATE THE RATE

1. There are _____ R waves in this 6-second strip.

2. This means the rate is _____ beats per minute.

3. Is this a normal rate? _____

9

90

yes

STEP 2. MEASURE THE REGULARITY OF THE R WAVES

1. Are the R-R intervals regular? _____

2. This means the ventricular rhythm can be classified as _____.

yes

regular

STEP 3. EXAMINE THE P WAVES

1. Are they of normal size and shape? _____

2. This means the pacemaker is in the _____ _____.

yes

SA node

STEP 4. MEASURE THE PR INTERVAL

1. What is the duration of the PR interval? _____.

2. Is this normal? _____

3. It means that there is a _____ in conduction.

4. At what site? Between the _____ and _____.

0.32 seconds
(8 squares × 0.04 seconds)

no

delay

atria, ventricles

STEP 5. MEASURE THE QRS COMPLEX

1. What is its duration? _____

2. Is this normal? _____

Now what have we learned from this strip?

1. The pacemaker is in the _____ _____.

2. There is normal _____ rhythm.

3. The PR interval is _____, indicating a _____
delay between the _____ and _____.

4. Conduction through the ventricles, however, is _____.

5. How do you know this? _____
_____.

6. What is the site of this conduction defect? _____ _____

7. Incidentally, the T waves are _____.

8. This may indicate _____ _____.

0.10 seconds

yes

SA node

sinus

prolonged, conduction
atria, ventricles

normal

the QRS duration is
normal (0.10 seconds)

AV node

inverted

myocardial ischemia

TERMINOLOGY REVIEW (*ICC, 4th ed., Chapter 8*)

Exercise 18

Complete the statements that follow the Word Rounds. If you wish to play Word Rounds, then locate your answer in the scrambled letters. Words are spelled from left to right and downward; there is one diagonal word. Circle your words.

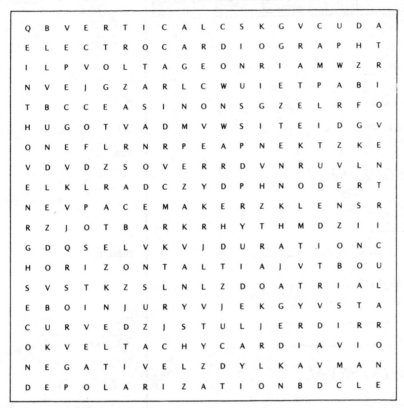

Figure 8.24. Word Rounds.

1. The instrument that detects electrical waves from the heart: _____.   electrocardiograph

2. Normal cardiac pacemaker: _____ node.   sinus

3. Positive deflection on ECG: _____.   upward

4. Small lines on ECG are _____ mm apart.   one

5. Voltage: _____.   amplitude

6. Arrhythmias due to disturbances of impulse formation may be classified by the sites of _____.   origin

7. Repolarization: _____.   recovery

8. Normal cardiac pacemaker (2 words): _____ _____.   SA node

9. The _____ where an arrhythmia began helps classify it.   site

10. "Battery" that discharges to cause heartbeat: _____.   pacemaker

11. The printed record of electrical waves from the heart: _____.   electrocardiogram

12. "Father of the electrocardiograph":   Einthoven

13. The _____ of His conducts the impulses from the AV node to the Purkinje fibers.   Bundle

14. 10 mm = _____ mv (on ECG).   one

15. The distance between_____ lines measures voltage on ECG.   horizontal

110

16. Arrhythmias originating outside the SA node but above the AV node are called _____ arrhythmias. | atrial

17. Normal PR should not be _____ 0.20 seconds (one word). | over

18. Heart rate over 100 per minute: _____. | tachycardia

19. Elevated or depressed ST segments may indicate muscle _____. | injury

20. Conduction _____ in the AV node prolongs the PR interval. | delay

21. Downward deflection on ECG: _____. | negative

22. Conduction of impulse through heart: _____. | depolarization

23. Another name for sinus node: _____-atrial. | sino

24. When impulses flow away from a positive electrode, the deflection on an ECG is _____. | downward

25. Bradycardia is a slow _____ arrhythmia. | rate

26. Amount of time measured from one _____ line to the next = 0.04 seconds (on ECG). | vertical

27. Time is measured on an ECG in fractions of a _____. | second

28. Intensity of electrical activity of the heart: _____. | voltage

29. By counting R waves, you can calculate heart _____. | rate

30. Island of specialized tissue in the conduction system of the heart: _____. | node

31. R waves in 6 seconds multiplied by _____ tells the minute rate. | ten

32. Amount of time required for conduction: _____. | duration

33. Normal Ps and Ts are _____ rather than pointed. | curved

34. _____body who can read a temperature graph can learn to read an ECG. | Any

35. Regularity of heartbeat: _____. | rhythm

The following abbreviations are also found in the Word Rounds:

1. Electrocardiogram, Anglicized: _____. | ECG

2. Electrocardiogram, German: _____. | EKG

3. Modified unipolar extremity lead (one of the 12 leads on an ECG): _____. | AVR

4. Rhythm all CCU nurses love: _____. | NSR

5. Segment on ECG that may change with injury to heart muscle: _____. | ST

6. Normal is 0.10 to 0.20 seconds: _____. | PR

7. From one R wave to the next R wave: _____. | RR

8. Node that has a slower inherent pacing rate than SA node: _____. | AV

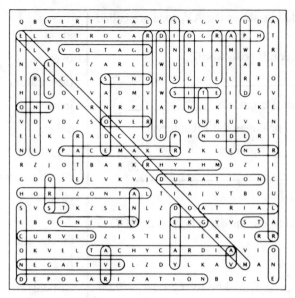

Figure 8.25. Answers to Word Rounds.

9

Arrhythmias Originating in the Sinoatrial (SA) Node

THE SA NODE (*ICC, 4th ed., p. 133*)

You've arrived! You're beginning to interpret arrhythmias. I hope you're excited and enthusiastic. First, perhaps we'd better get oriented; we're going to start at the top of the heart and work down. In other words, we'll start at the beginning of the conduction system (the SA node) and study arrhythmias that arise there. Then we'll work downward to the atria, the AV node, and the ventricles. In general, the severity of arrhythmias increases as we descend. You'll soon see what I mean.

Exercise 1

1. You already know that the normal pacemaker is the _____ _____.

   SA node

2. Normal sinus rate is _____ to _____ beats per minute.

   60, 100

3. However, the SA node can discharge_____ or_____ than 60-100.

   faster, slower

4. The SA node's rate is affected by the _____ and _____ nervous systems.

   sympathetic
   parasympathetic

5. Increased sympathetic stimulation (speeds/slow) the heart.

   speeds

6. Increased parasympathetic stimulation (speed/slows) the heart.

   slows

7. The electrical discharge of the SA node is shown by the_____ wave on an ECG.

   P

8. Arrhythmias arising from the sinus node are characterized by abnormal rates of the _____ waves.

   P

SINUS TACHYCARDIA (*ICC, 4th ed., pp. 134-135*)

In studying each arrhythmia, be sure you understand the identifying ECG features that accompany the ECGs in Chapter 9, *ICC*, 4th ed. When you come to the examples,

113

cover the interpretations and try to complete them for yourself. This will give you some practice along with ready answers.

Exercise 2

1. With sinus tachycardia, the pacemaker is the ____ _____. — SA node

2. The rate is usually between _____ and _____ beats per minute. — 100, 150

3. Increased stimulation of the SA node by the _____ nervous system is usually the cause of this arrhythmia. — sympathetic

4. This overactivity is usually a reaction to _____, _____, or _____. — fever, anxiety activity

5. If after running around the block your pulse is 120/minute, you probably have _____ _____. — sinus tachycardia

6. Sinus tachycardia usually terminates (suddenly/gradually). — gradually

7. This (is/is not) a dangerous arrhythmia in its own right. — is not

8. The danger lies in the _____ _____ of the arrhythmia. — underlying cause

9. If it is due to fever, it may be treated with _____. — aspirin

10. If caused by anxiety, it may be treated with _____. — tranquilizers

11. A nurse who recognizes the faces of fear may be able to help by giving the patient _____ or _____ support. — psychological, emotional

12. The most serious cause of sinus tachycardia is _____ _____ _____. — left ventricular failure

13. In this case, _____ may be helpful. — digitalis

14. Careful nursing observation can help in determining the _____ of sinus tachycardia. — cause

SINUS BRADYCARDIA (ICC, 4th ed., pp. 136-137)

Exercise 3

1. The pacemaker is the _____ _____. — SA node

2. The rate is usually between _____ and _____. — 40, 60

3. Increased stimulation by the _____ nervous system is often the cause. — parasympathetic

4. Or, a phrase you'll hear many times: Excess _____ stimulation slows the SA node. — vagal

5. The rate is slow, but each normal QRS is preceded by a normal _____. — P wave

Now things get a bit more complicated, and I'd like to try a little "tea party" to simplify them. Suppose we compare the pacemaker cells of the heart's conduction system to a group of ladies at an afternoon tea. Mrs. SA Node, who talks the fastest, usually dominates the conversation. She's the normal pacesetter. However, if she tires and slows down, her sister-in-law, Mrs. Junctional, takes over. If all the others run down, slow-speaking Mrs. Ventricle may control the conversation. Then, too, one of the slower ladies can suddenly become fired up over a topic and dominate the conversation.

Thus, the various pacemaker cells of the conduction system have the potential to take over as pacemaker for the heart under certain conditions. Or, failing to assume control, they can still impose themselves and interfere with regular rhythm. Pacemakers from ectopic foci (abnormal sites) are a possibility any time the basic rate of the heart becomes too slow.

While the tea cools, try these:

6. If the sinus node_____ to below 60 per minute, other cells (ectopic foci) may pace the heart.

   slows

7. Ectopic arrhythmias, especially ventricular, (are/are not) dangerous.

   are

8. A significant decrease in heart rate can cause a_____ in cardiac output.

   decrease

9. Severely decreased cardiac output reduces the blood supply to the _____ and arteries of the _____.

   brain
   heart

10. Sinus bradycardia should be considered a (lethal/warning/benign) arrhythmia.

   warning

11. Uncomplicated sinus bradycardia will probably (be/not be) treated.

   not be

12. Sinus bradycardia is usually treated only if it causes_____ or _____.

   symptoms
   complications

13. Can you list the 3 indications for treatment of sinus bradycardia?
_____
_____
_____

   if ventricular ectopic beats occur
   if cardiac output falls
   if the heart rate is less than 50

14. If the doctor does treat this arrhythmia, he'll probably try_____ first.

   atropine

15. Dosage will probably be _____ to _____.

   0.5, 1.0 mg

16. Mode of administration will be _____.

   intravenously

17. If atropine fails, _____ (trade name) may be given by IV drip.

   Isuprel

18. The generic name for this drug is _____.

   isoproterenol

19. If drug treatments fail and symptoms are severe, _____ _____ may be tried to speed the heart rate.

   transvenous
   pacing

20. Can you list some drugs you might "hold" while you call the doctor if your patient develops bradycardia? _____, _____, _____, _____.

   reserpine, digitalis
   morphine, propranolol

21. If the heart rate is less than 60 per minute, you can assume sinus bradycardia is present. (True/False)

   False

22. All sinus rhythms must have a _____ wave preceding every normal QRS.

   P

23. So you'd check the ECG carefully for_____ waves. (No P waves? This bradycardia is not sinus. It could be more dangerous: notify the doctor.)

   P

24. If the heart rate falls below _____ per minute, call the doctor.

   50

25. Suppose atropine is given. You'd watch the heart _____ carefully to see if it speeds up.

   rate

26. If Isuprel is ordered, you'd give it (slowly/rapidly) IV drip.
Isuprel is like fire—a good friend or a lethal weapon. Run it slowly, increase it slowly, check the blood pressure frequently, and watch for increased ectopic activity.

   slowly

SINUS ARRHYTHMIA (ICC, 4th ed., pp. 138-139)

Have you ever taken a pulse that cycles faster and then slower in a rhythmic pattern? Very likely your own does. This is a "normal" arrhythmia—important because we must distinguish it from dangerous arrhythmia.

Exercise 4

1. Sinus arrhythmia (is/is not) a dangerous arrhythmia.

   is not

2. It (is/is not) a warning arrhythmia.

   is not

3. It (should/should not) be treated.
   should not

4. Usually the heart rate (decreases/increases) with inspiration.
   increases

WANDERING PACEMAKER (*ICC, 4th ed., pp. 140-141*)

Exercise 5

1. The pacemaker may wander within the _____ node.
   SA

2. Or the pacemaker may wander away from the _____ node.
   SA

3. It may wander to the _____ _____.
   junctional area

4. The only means of diagnosis is by _____.
   ECG

5. The only ECG evidence is a change in the configuration of the _____ waves.
   P

6. This (is/is not) a dangerous or a warning arrhythmia.
   is not

7. Treatment (is/is not) required.
   is not

8. But you should watch the monitor to be sure that the _____ foci do not assume full control.
   ectopic

9. This arrhythmia probably results from increased _____ influence.
   vagal

SINUS ARREST (*ICC, 4th ed., pp. 142-143*)

Exercise 6

"Hey, Nurse, my heart just skipped a beat." The monitor gives you the information, too—a missing PQRS and T. It is not a serious problem unless the "skipping" is frequent or consecutive—then watch out!

1. The terms *sinus arrest* and *sinus block* are generally used interchangeably. (True/False)
   True

2. In sinus arrest, the sinus node _____ to fire an impulse.
   fails

3. Or the impulse is _____ within the SA node (sinus block).
   blocked

4. In either case, would you see a P wave for that interval?
   no

5. Would you see a QRS wave for that interval? _____
   no

6. The ECG shows no _____ _____ for one beat.
   PQRST complex

7. The usual cause is (decreased/increased) vagal influence.
   increased

8. _____ toxicity may cause sinus arrest.
   Digitalis

9. A more dangerous cause may be _____ of the SA node.
   ischemia

10. Repeated or consecutive dropped beats can lead to _____ cardiac output.
   decreased

11. Symptoms of decreased cardiac output you should watch for are _____, _____, _____, and _____ _____.
   hypotension, syncope, angina, heart failure

Exercise 7

Let's say your patient, Mr. Kardiak, is having sinus arrest for one beat a few times an hour.

1. On the monitor you'd note a _____ complex.
   missing

2. You'd better _____ the arrhythmia on a rhythm strip.
   document or record

3. You'd watch the monitor to see if the frequency of these missed beats _____.

increases

4. Now it's time for Mr. Kardiak to have his digitalis. What do you do? _____
_____
_____.

Hold the digitalis and ask if the doctor wants it given

5. You notice that the periods of sinus arrest are becoming more frequent. The doctor will probably order _____. Dosage? _____ to _____ _____.

atropine, 0.5, 1 mg, IV

6. If this doesn't work _____ may be tried.

Isuprel

7. If drug therapy doesn't work _____ _____ may be necessary.

transvenous pacing

8. Frequent sinus arrest is a (serious-warning/lethal) arrhythmia.

serious-warning

REVIEW (*ICC, 4th ed., Chapter 9*)

We've covered 5 different types of arrhythmias so far. By now you should know how to identify them, what their dangers are, how to treat them, and what to do when they develop. Let's see how you've progressed.

Exercise 8

I've prepared a list of short statements that relate to one *or more* of the arrhythmias. Match the statements with the 5 arrhythmias. Some are easy, but others will challenge you. We'll give each of the arrhythmias a letter to simplify things.

　　　　　A. Sinus Tachycardia
　　　　　B. Sinus Bradycardia
　　　　　C. Sinus Arrhythmia
　　　　　D. SA Block
　　　　　E. Wandering Pacemaker

_____ 1. one full cardiac cycle is missing	D
_____ 2. AV node may take over	E
_____ 3. hold digitalis	B, D
_____ 4. cyclic pattern	C
_____ 5. digitalis may help	A
_____ 6. may result from morphine	B
_____ 7. caused by ischemia of SA	D
_____ 8. abnormal P waves, normal QRSs	E
_____ 9. rate increases with inspiration	C
_____ 10. may be due to fever	A
_____ 11. stops gradually	A
_____ 12. patient may feel faint	B, D
_____ 13. not dangerous at all	C
_____ 14. may require atropine	B, D, E
_____ 15. rate changes with breath holding	C
_____ 16. P waves vary in configuration	E
_____ 17. may be due to vagal overactivity	B, D, E
_____ 18. may cause reduction in cardiac output	B, D
_____ 19. potentially dangerous if frequent	D

_____ 20. recognized only on ECG   E

_____ 21. may require cardiac pacing   B, D

_____ 22. dropped beat   D

_____ 23. rate decreases with expiration   C

_____ 24. may be due to left ventricular failure A

_____ 25. never produces symptoms   C

_____ 26. hold quinidine   B, D

_____ 27. ectopic pacemaker may take over   B, D, E

_____ 28. R-R time varies over 0.12 seconds   C

_____ 29. aberrant P waves   E

Congratulations! You're doing excellent work.

MONITOR PRACTICE (*ICC, 4th ed., Chapter 9*)

Exercise 9

Let's take a look at some patients on the monitors. Fill in the blanks and answer the questions.

Patient: *Mr. Big Builder*
Diagnosis: Acute MI

Mr. BB's brother and partner in the electrical contracting business visits him. They discuss their heavy workload and contracts they may lose while BB is hospitalized. The high rate alarm rings on BB's monitor, and you see the following pattern on his scope.

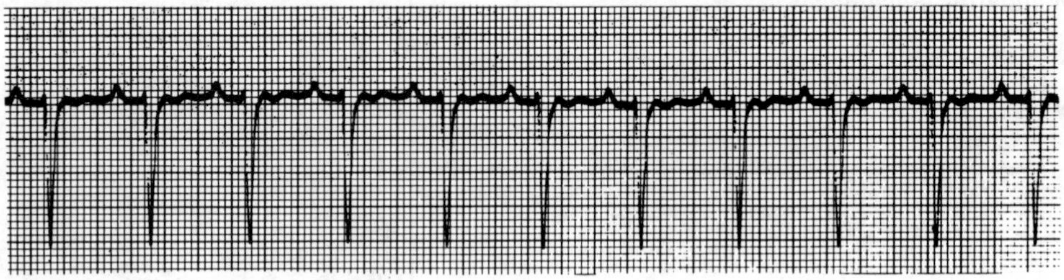

Figure 9.1.

1. Arrhythmia diagnosis: _____ _____   sinus tachycardia

2. Probable cause: _____nervous system stimulation due to   sympathetic anxiety
   _____.

3. What nursing action would you take in this situation?   A, possibly B & C

   A. Call partner out of room and explain his talk is upsetting BB.

   B. Tell partner visiting time is up, and he must leave.

   C. Give BB his prn tranquilizer.

   D. Tell BB he needs to relax and stop worrying.

Think out the pros and cons of each of these choices, then read the discussion that follows.

Discussion of Nursing Action (*Question 3*)

A. Partner may not understand or cooperate; however, with some visitors it may work. Partner may then put on an act of "everything is fine." BB knows better and will worry more. BB may be upset and suspicious because you called his visitor out.

118

How well do you know your patient and his visitors? Could you handle him this way?

B. If this isn't true, both BB and his partner will know it. If true, it should be done tactfully and courteously. BB may continue to worry and imagine worse problems than actually exist.

C. He may make a determined effort to resist the tranquilizer's effect in order to continue his business.

D. Ineffective. If he could relax, he would.

Correct nursing action may be a combination of A, possibly B, and C. It depends on your knowledge of Mr. BB. After the partner leaves, give BB a chance to talk while you give him a back rub and the tranquilizer takes effect. Two phrases you might use: "Do you want to talk about it?" and "It must be tough to. . . ."

Exercise 10

Patient: *Mr. Kardiak*
Diagnosis: Acute MI

This man had an MI about 20 hours ago. He has taken reserpine for hypertension for 6 months. In the hospital the orders also include morphine every 4 hours, prn, potassium two times a day, and digitalis once a day. You note the following ECG on his monitor.

Answers and discussion follow.

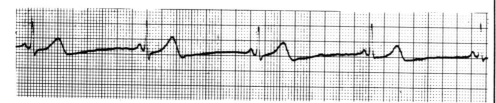

Figure 9.2.

1. Arrhythmia diagnosis: _____ _____
   > sinus bradycardia

2. Probable cause: parasympathetic nervous system (_____) dominance of the _____ _____.
   > vagal
   > SA node

3. Should you withhold drugs ordered? (Yes/No)
   If so, which drugs? _____, _____, _____.
   > Yes
   > reserpine, morphine, digitalis

4. Notify doctor? (Yes/No)
   > Yes

5. Which drugs would you have ready for possible treatment? _____, _____.
   > Atropine
   > Isuprel

6. What other treatment might be needed if rate remains too slow? _____ _____.
   > Transvenous
   > pacing

7. Would you administer morphine if he complained of chest pain? (Yes/No)
   > NO, don't administer morphine

8. The most likely treatment for this arrhythmia would be:

   _____
   (drug)   (dose)   (mode of administration)
   > The doctor would probably first try atropine, 0.5 to 1.0 mg, IV

9. After the first drug fails, the doctor orders isoproterenol. What brand name might you find it under? _____
   > Isuprel

The Head Nurse mixes and hangs the isoproterenol drip (you're not sure of the concentration), sets it at 10 drops per minute, and goes to lunch.

Mr. Kardiak's heart rate doesn't increase after 10 minutes. Would you:

10. Increase IV to 20 drops per minute?

Don't you dare increase the IV rate to 20 drops!

11. Increase IV by 2 drops every 2 to 5 minutes?

An increase of 2 drops every 2 to 5 minutes would be ok *IF* you knew the concentration you were using. But you don't know.

12. Find out the concentration of IV and label it?

Definitely

13. Call the doctor?

Yes. I'd call the doctor. You'd certainly expect the rate to increase with isoproteronol. Something doesn't seem right.

10

Arrhythmias Originating in the Atria

Ready now to move out from the sinus node and learn about the arrhythmias coming from the atria?

Exercise 1 (*ICC, 4th ed., p. 147*)

1. You know that the _____ _____ is the normal pacemaker of the heart.

   SA node

2. This is because it normally discharges at a (faster/slower) rate than any other area of the heart.

   faster

3. Is it possible for the SA node to be depressed and fire slower than usual? _____

   yes

4. Is it possible for an ectopic focus to become irritable and fire faster than the SA node? _____

   yes

5. What happens then? _____

   the ectopic focus can take over

6. If the ectopic focus (or foci) is in the atria, an _____ arrhythmia develops.

   atrial

7. Atrial ectopic foci can take over for only _____ beat, or they can take over _____.

   one
   continuously

8. If atrial impulses occur at rates of less than 200 per minute, P waves can usually be seen. (True/False)

   True

9. However, the P waves are usually _____ in shape,

   distorted

10. because the pacemaker is not in the _____ _____.

    SA node

Exercise 2

Remember, it's the atria that are contracting at fantastically rapid rates; the ventricles can't contract that fast and still manage to fill and pump out blood. So the AV node protects the ventricles from what could be serious rapidity. Now try these:

1. With very fast atrial rates, the AV node protects the ventricles by _____ some of the atrial impulses.

   blocking

2. With atrial rates under 200 per minute, the AV node usually (does/does not) block atrial impulses.

does not

3. Thus, each P wave would be followed by a _____.

QRS

4. With atrial rates of 200-400, the AV node may _____ some, but not all, of the atrial impulses.

block

5. Thus, there will be (more/fewer) P waves than QRS waves.

more

6. With atrial rates much over 400 per minute, the atria simply _____ because they can't respond to so many stimuli.

twitch

7. This is called _____ _____.

atrial fibrillation

8. In this case, impulses reach the AV node irregularly, so conduction to the ventricles is _____ too.

irregular

9. As a result, the ventricular rhythm becomes _____.

irregular

10. Thus, in atrial arrhythmias the ventricular rate and rhythm are determined by the number of _____ impulses and whether they are blocked at the _____ _____.

atrial, AV node

Exercise 3

Although *ICC*, 4th ed., p. 147, stresses the danger of atrial arrhythmias, it is important to realize that some people live all their lives with these conditions. So let's discuss the etiology of atrial arrhythmias and find out just when they are dangerous.

1. Irritability of atrial cells is usually due to _____ or _____ _____.

ischemia, atrial overdistention

2. This irritability leads to atrial _____.

arrhythmias

3. Atrial arrhythmias can cause the ventricular rate to _____ greatly.

increase

4. Very rapid ventricular rates can cause a _____ in cardiac output.

decrease

5. Why? _____

because the time for ventricular filling is shortened

6. These atrial arrhythmias would be considered _____ arrhythmias if they occurred after an MI.

dangerous or major

7. If a patient has been in normal sinus rhythm before an MI and develops atrial arrhythmias after an MI, these (should/should not) be treated.

should

8. Why? _____

because they may reduce cardiac output

9. If a patient has lived with atrial fibrillation for years before an MI, the atrial arrhythmia probably (does/does not) have to be treated (except to control rapid ventricular rates.)

does not

10. The great danger of atrial arrhythmias is the fast _____ rate they may produce.

ventricular

PREMATURE ATRIAL CONTRACTION
(*ICC, 4th ed., pp. 148-149*)

I'd like to introduce you to the triplets, PAC, PNC, and PVC. PAC is probably the least troublesome of the three. You'll meet the other two later.

Exercise 4

1. A premature baby comes _____ he is expected.

before

2. Premature beats come _____ the normal beat is expected.

before

3. A premature beat is an (ectopic/normal) beat. | ectopic

4. Ectopic beats can come from _____ areas (foci) in the heart. | irritable

5. PACs come from irritable foci in the _____. | atria

6. The patient usually (does/does not) feel these beats. | does not

7. PACs are diagnosed by _____. | ECG

8. You (would/would not) see a P wave with a PAC. | would

9. The configuration of the P wave with a PAC (would/would not) be normal. | would not

10. PACs (are/are not) inherently dangerous. | are not

11. PACs may warn of increasing atrial _____. | irritability

12. The most frequently used treatment for excessive PACs: _____ and/or _____. | digitalis quinidine

13. Can PACs cause an irregular pulse? _____ | yes, if frequent

I'd like to give you a hint on how to check an ECG for regularity of the heartbeat. Sometimes you can't be sure by simply looking at the R waves, and you need a more exact method. One way of doing this is to use measuring calipers, which should be part of the equipment in a CCU. But since you might not carry these with you, all you have to do is lay a piece of scrap paper across the rhythm strip so that the R waves show above it. Now make marks on the scrap paper where the first 3 R waves appear. Then slide the paper to the right so that the mark on the first R wave is now on the third R wave. If the rhythm is regular, the marks will fall directly on succeeding R waves. If they don't, you know the rhythm is irregular.

Try this method on the following ECG. Is the rhythm regular or irregular? | irregular

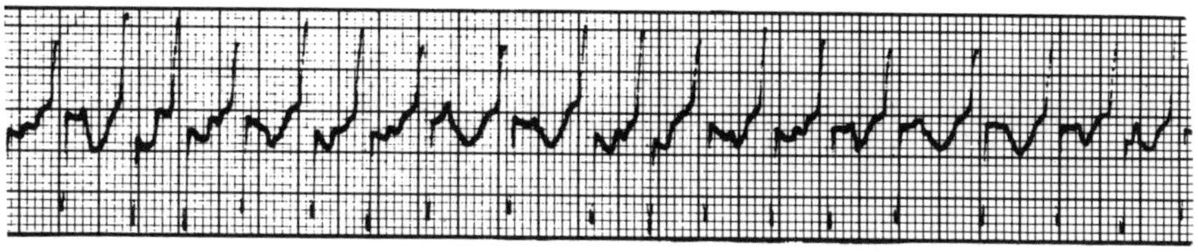

Figure 10.1.

PAROXYSMAL ATRIAL TACHYCARDIA
(*ICC, 4th ed., pp. 150-151*)

You've just learned that in PAC the P stands for "premature," but in PAT the P means "paroxysmal." Look the word up if necessary; you'll use it a lot.

Exercise 5

1. A tachycardia is a continuous heart rate over _____ per minute. | 100

2. The T in PAT stands for _____. | tachycardia

3. Paroxysmal means to start and stop _____. | suddenly

4. Sinus tachycardia is usually paroxysmal. (True/False) | False

5. Atrial tachycardia is usually paroxysmal. (True/False) | True

6. The atrial rate in PAT is usually _____ to _____ per minute. | 150, 250

7. The ventricular rate in PAT is usually _____ to _____ per minute. | 150, 250

8. PAT is caused by an irritable _____ _____. | atrial focus

9. Patients usually (can/cannot) feel PAT. | can

10. A rapid PAT can (increase/decrease) cardiac output. | decrease

123

11. Decreased cardiac output can cause _____ _____ _____.	left ventricular failure
12. Rapid ventricular rates can (increase/decrease) myocardial oxygen demand.	increase
13. Increased demand and decreased output can cause myocardial _____.	ischemia
14. Myocardial ischemia can cause _____.	angina
15. After an MI, PAT (is/is not) dangerous.	is
16. The longer PAT lasts, the _____ the danger.	greater
17. PAT can sometimes be stopped by pressure on the _____ or the _____. (Sometimes this works too well; I wouldn't try it alone without a definite order.)	carotid sinuses eyeballs
18. Asymptomatic PAT can be treated with _____ or _____- _____ _____ or _____.	morphine, rapid-acting digitalis, propranolol
19. To prevent recurrences of PAT, _____, orally, is often effective.	quinidine
20. If PAT persists, elective precordial _____ should be given.	shock

ATRIAL FLUTTER (*ICC, 4th ed., pp. 152-153*)

Look at the example strip on page 153 of *ICC*, 4th ed. This is classically described as a "sawtoothed" pattern.

Exercise 6

1. In atrial flutter, the pacemaker is an ectopic focus in the _____.	atria
2. The rate of this atrial focus is _____ to _____ per minute.	250, 400
3. The AV node protects the ventricle from this rapid rate by _____ some of the atrial impulses.	blocking
4. True P waves are replaced by _____ waves.	flutter
5. There are (more/fewer) flutter waves than QRSs.	more
6. Generally you can count out a ratio of _____ waves to _____ waves.	atrial or flutter ventricular
7. There may be a 2:1, 3:1, 4:1 atrial/ventricular _____.	block
8. The patient's block (can/cannot) change.	can
9. If it changes, the ventricular rate will be (regular/irregular).	irregular
10. You already know that rapid ventricular rates decrease _____ _____.	cardiac output
11. and cause myocardial _____ and _____.	ischemia, angina
12. Atrial flutter is a dangerous arrhythmia if the ventricular rate is _____.	rapid
13. The surest treatment for atrial flutter is _____ _____.	synchronized shock
14. Thought question: Your patient is in atrial flutter with a ventricular rate of about 80. He's in no discomfort. Why would you monitor him closely?	Atrial flutter blocks are variable; his ventricular rate can change at any time if the AV block changes.

ATRIAL FIBRILLATION (*ICC, 4th ed., pp. 154-157*)

A doctor once told me, "Nurses misdiagnose atrial fibrillation more often than any other type of arrhythmia." Since we see a great deal of it, we'll concentrate on learning to diagnose it correctly.

Exercise 7

1. In atrial fibrillation, the pacemaker is an ectopic focus (or foci) in the _____.
atria

2. The atrial rate is over _____ per minute.
400

3. The AV node is bombarded by these atrial impulses; it conducts (regularly/irregularly) to the ventricles.
irregularly

4. If the ventricular response is over 100 per minute, it's called _____ atrial fibrillation.
rapid

5. If the ventricular rate is below 100 per minute, it's called _____ atrial fibrillation.
slow

6. Rapid ventricular rates _____ the threat of left ventricular failure.
increase

7. The apical (heart) rate is usually (more/less) than the radial (pulse) rate.
more

8. Thus, if an unmonitored patient has a totally irregular pulse, you should take the _____ rate.
apical

9. The difference between apical and radial pulse is called _____ _____.
pulse deficit

10. Finding a pulse deficit on an unmonitored patient with an irregular pulse might make you suspect he has _____ _____.
atrial fibrillation

11. The atria (do/do not) contract in atrial fibrillation.
do not

12. The loss of atrial contraction _____ ventricular filling.
reduces or decreases

13. Decreased ventricular filling may also contribute to left ventricular _____, and myocardial _____.
failure
ischemia

14. Blood clots tend to form in the noncontracting _____.
atria

15. Uncontrolled atrial fibrillation (is/is not) a dangerous arrhythmia when it occurs after an MI.
is

16. Atrial fibrillation that is causing complications should be terminated with _____ _____.
synchronized shock

17. If atrial fibrillation is treated with drugs, _____ is given to increase the AV block.
digitalis

18. Increasing the AV block with digitalis helps to _____ the ventricular rate.
slow or decrease

19. Atrial fibrillation can sometimes be converted to normal sinus rhythm with drugs, especially _____.
quinidine

On the ECG there are two hallmarks of atrial fibrillation: an irregular, indefinable baseline (a "messy" baseline), and total irregularity of the R waves. Remember these two, and please note: the ventricular rate and/or width of the QRS is not part of the criteria for diagnosis of atrial fibrillation.

ATRIAL STANDSTILL (*ICC, 4th ed., pp. 158-159*)

Exercise 8

Look at the rhythm strip on page 159 of *ICC*, 4th ed. Can you find any P waves? (I hope not!) As you know, the P waves show depolarization of the atria, and obviously these atria are just sitting there—or standing there.

1. The normal pacemaker is the _____ _____.
SA node

2. If it fails, we hope the _____ will generate impulses.
atria

3. Sudden loss of P waves on the monitor can be a warning of impending atrial _____.
standstill

125

4. With loss of atrial activity, the pacemaker descends to the _____ _____ or (junctional) area.

AV nodal

5. Failure of the junctional area leaves only the _____ pacemakers to initiate impulses.

ventricular

6. This progression is called _____ displacement of the pacemaker.

downward

7. Downward displacement may be associated with left _____ _____ or cardiogenic _____.

ventricular failure, shock

8. Overdosages of _____ and _____ can cause downward displacement of the pacemaker.

digitalis, quinidine

9. Electrolyte imbalances, _____, can also cause atrial standstill.

hyperkalemia

10. However, the usual cause is irreversible damage to higher _____ centers.

pacemaker

11. Atrial standstill is an ominous warning of progressive _____ _____ of the pacemaker.

downward displacement

12. Lower pacemaker centers are inherently (slower/faster) and (less/just as) reliable than higher centers.

slower, less

13. Primary treatment is to institute _____ _____.

transvenous pacing

MONITOR PRACTICE (*ICC, 4th ed., Chapter 10*)

Exercise 9

It seems to me that atrial arrhythmias are more interesting than any of the others. They're less lethal than ventricular arrhythmias, and some of them look downright pretty on the monitor. All of the following example strips are from patients who had MIs. Fill in the answers.

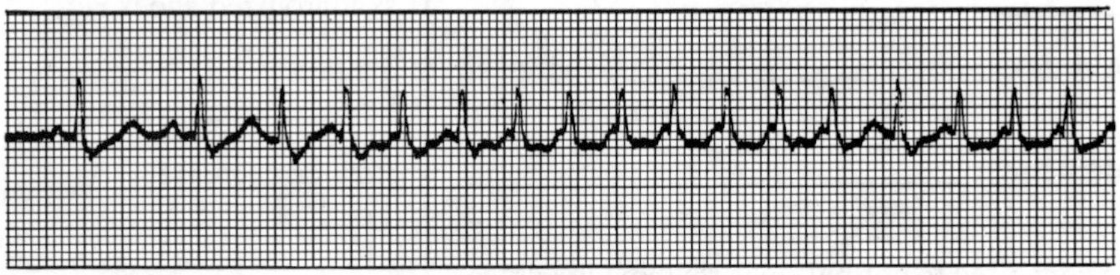

Figure 10.2. Mr. Whoops

It's breakfast time in CCU. Things are quiet, when suddenly the high-rate alarm rings.

1. The first two beats originate in the _____ _____.

SA node

2. Then, whoops! He develops _____ _____ _____.

paroxysmal atrial tachycardia

3. The rapid rate may cause _____.

angina

4. If sustained, it may lead to _____ _____ _____.

left ventricular failure

5. Would you observe this arrhythmia for a few minutes, or call the doctor stat? Why?
_____
_____
_____

Observe for a few minutes. It may stop spontaneously. Besides, you want to see if the patient develops any symptoms with the tachycardia.

6. This is a lethal arrhythmia. (True/False)

False

126

7. If this arrhythmia recurs, you would anticipate using which of the following: atropine, rapid-acting digitalis, Isuprel, or transvenous pacing?

rapid-acting digitalis

Exercise 10

He was just admitted, and has no symptoms now. You take an admission rhythm strip and see the following ECG. Insignificant looking, isn't it? Or is it? Better look carefully.

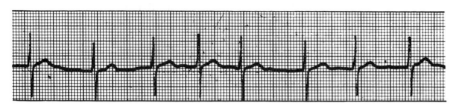

Figure 10.3. Mr. Ho-Hum

1. Are P waves present and normal? _____

No P waves are present

2. What does that tell you? _____

The pacemaker is *not* in the SA node

3. Are the R-R times regular? _____

No, they're irregular

4. No P waves and totally irregular R-R = _____ _____

atrial fibrillation

5. What is the ventricular rate? _____

80 per minute

6. Is this rapid atrial fibrillation? _____

No, it's slow, since ventricular rate is less than 100 per minute

7. Should you document the arrhythmia? _____

yes

8. Should you call the doctor stat? _____

No, this isn't an emergency. Call the doctor after you have all the admission information

9. You would want to ask the patient if he has been taking _____.

digitalis

10. What is the most important factor in deciding whether the arrhythmia should be treated? _____

whether or not the patient has left ventricular failure

11. Could this arrhythmia have been present for many years and not be related to myocardial infarction? _____

Yes. Many patients have atrial fibrillation. And it may have no connection with the acute MI

Exercise 11

The QRS complexes are inverted because of the position of the chest electrodes.

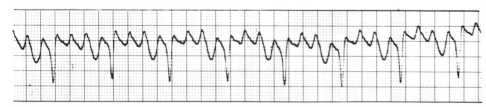

Figure 10.4. Ms. Rick-Rack

1. ECG interpretation: _____ _____.

atrial flutter

2. The atrial focus is discharging at a rate of _____ per minute (or _____ flutter waves in _____ seconds).

320, 32

6

3. The ventricular rate is _____. | 80 per minute

4. This means the _____ node is blocking some atrial impulses to protect the ventricle. | AV

5. What is the ratio of flutter waves (F waves) to R waves: _____ | 4:1

6. Are the R-R times regular? _____ | yes

7. Would they be in atrial fibrillation? _____ _____ | No, they'd be irregular in atrial fibrillation

8. The doctor may order a rapid-acting type of _____ _____. | digitalis preparation

9. Perhaps the most effective treatment for this arrhythmia is _____ _____. | precordial shock (cardioversion)

10. This is usually successful even with very _____ energy settings. | low

Exercise 12

He's been in the CCU for 2 days. He has had signs of mild left ventricular failure, but no digitalis has been given. Today he developed this arrhythmia.

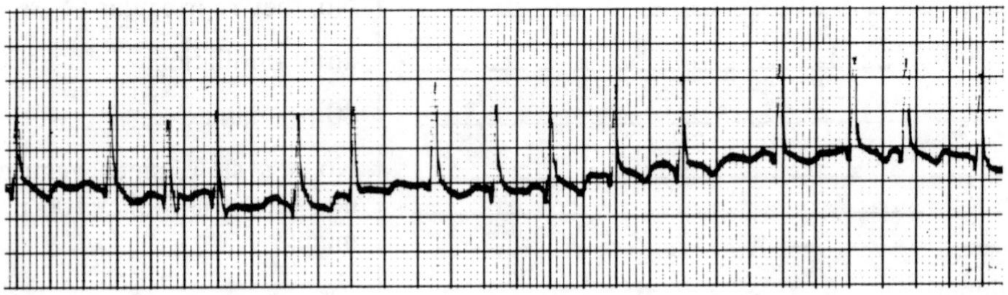

Figure 10.5. Mr. A.F.

1. What is the ventricular rate? _____. | 150 per minute

2. Is the rhythm regular? _____. | No, it's irregular

3. Is the baseline regular? _____. | No, the baseline varies

4. ECG diagnosis: _____ . _____. | atrial fibrillation

5. Is the ventricular rate "slow"? _____. | No, it's rapid

6. This arrhythmia may _____ the pumping efficiency of the heart. | decrease

7. Since the patient already has left ventricular failure, it may get _____. | worse

8. Treatment might include _____, which slows the ventricular rate. | digitalis

9. It is possible that the arrhythmia could be converted to normal sinus rhythm by means of _____ _____ _____. | synchronized precordial shock (cardioversion)

Now that you've interpreted the rhythm strips, draw a big breath. You've completed sinus and atrial arrhythmias and should be quite proud of yourself.

11

Arrhythmias Originating in the AV Nodal Area

JUNCTIONAL ARRHYTHMIAS (*ICC, 4th ed., p. 163*)

Medical and nursing knowledge must be continually updated as we learn more about that most fascinating species—the human. Chapter 11, *ICC,* 4th ed., introduces some new concepts and terms pertaining to arrhythmias originating in the AV nodal area. If you learned older terminology, i.e., AV nodal arrhythmias, try some simple updating and substitute the term *junctional* for AV nodal. (Of course, that isn't all there is to it.) And then let's update our knowledge to go with our new terminology.

Exercise 1

1. The AV node (does/does not) initiate impulses.   does not

2. The area around the AV node is called the _____ area.   junctional

3. The junctional area (can/cannot) initiate impulses.   can

4. Thus, arrhythmias originating in the AV nodal area are called _____ arrhythmias.   junctional

5. The junctional area's inherent discharge rate is (slower/faster) than the SA node.   slower

6. If the junctional area takes over as pacemaker, you'd expect a rate of about _____ to _____ per minute.   40, 60

7. This would be called a _____ rhythm or a junctional _____ rhythm.   junctional / escape

8. Junctional rhythms occur when _____ pacing centers are depressed.   higher

9. Increased activity of the junctional area can lead to faster _____ rhythms (above 60/min.).   junctional

10. In general, rapid rates are called _____.   tachycardias

11. A tachycardia that starts and stops suddenly is called a _____ tachycardia.   paroxysmal

129

12. A fast-rate arrhythmia originating paroxysmally in the junctional tissue would be called _____ junctional tachycardia.

paroxysmal

13. If the tachycardia began gradually, it could be termed non-_____ juntional tachycardia (NPJT).

(non)-paroxysmal

14. Another name for NPJT is _____ _____ _____.

accelerated junctional rhythm

15. Ectopic premature beats originating from around AV nodal area are called _____ _____ _____, abbreviated as _____.

premature junctional contractions, PJC

16. If the SA node and atria fail to discharge impulses, downward displacement of the pacemaker occurs and the _____ _____ is next in line to serve as pacemaker.

junctional area

17. This could happen after _____ to the higher centers.

injury or ischemia

18. Thus, junctional arrhythmias (except PJCs) are considered (major/minor) arrhythmias.

major

PREMATURE JUNCTIONAL CONTRACTIONS
(*ICC, 4th ed., pp. 164-165*)

Exercise 2

How about some What, Where, Why, When questions? Let's start off with the cause of PJC.

1. An ectopic focus in the _____ area can initiate an impulse _____ the SA impulse.

      where
    when

junctional
before

2. This stimulus is transmitted _____ through the _____ system and produces ventricular _____.

    where   *what*
    what

downward, His-Purkinje
depolarization

3. The ectopic junctional impulse can also go _____ and _____ the atria.

    where   *what*

upward depolarize

4. If atrial depolarization precedes ventricular depolarization, you'll see a _____ before the QRS on the ECG.

    what

P wave

5. If atrial and ventricular depolarization are simultaneous, the _____ can be "buried" in the _____ and not be visible.

    what
    what

P wave
QRS

6. If the atria depolarize *after* the ventricles, on the ECG you'll see a _____ wave first and then a _____.

QRS
P wave

7. Since atrial depolarization is from the "bottom up" or retrograde, the P waves may appear _____ (or "upside down").

    how

inverted

8. PJCs are caused by _____ of the junctional tissue, probably due to _____.

    what
    what

irritability
ischemia

9. PJCs (are/are not) considered serious or major arrhythmias.

are not

Exercise 3

Ms. Pre Junque is a 95-pound, 85-year-old antique dealer, a post-MI in your unit. You begin noticing premature ectopic beats on the monitor. What would you do?

1. _____ the arrhythmia by running a rhythm strip.

Document

2. _____ the patient's clinical status by inquiring how she feels. ("Just fine, Honey, just fine.")

Assess

3. _____ her vital signs ("Y'all gonna wear my poor ole arm out, Honey.") | Check

4. Study the monitor strip, looking especially at the relationship of _____ waves and _____ complexes. | P QRS

5. It's important to differentiate PJCs from _____. | PVCs

6. If you aren't sure whether it is a PVC or PJC, you may need to get a ____-_____ _____. | 12-lead ECG

7. While Ms. Junque raves about the market for antique shoehorns, you continue to evaluate the situation: The ectopics are increasing. You get ready to administer either _____ IV or _____ and then call the doctor. | lidocaine, procainamide

JUNCTIONAL RHYTHM (*ICC, 4th ed., pp. 166-167*)

Exercise 4

When higher pacemakers are depressed, the junctional area can take over at rates below 60 per minute and pace the heart. Is this a problem? Does it make any difference who pitches, as long as we have a ball game? Suppose we think this through.

1. In junctional rhythm the pacemaker is in the _____ _____. | junctional tissue

2. It paces at a rate of about _____ to _____ beats per minute. | 40, 60

3. Junctional rhythm is possible when the SA node is _____. | depressed

4. The SA node may be depressed due to increased _____ stimulation. | vagal

5. Other causes of SA depression may be _____ or overdoses of _____ or _____. | ischemia, digitalis quinidine

6. Junctional rhythm can only be diagnosed for certain by _____. | ECG

7. Junctional rhythm is often (temporary/permanent). | temporary

8. However, any slow rhythm is dangerous because of _____ cardiac output. | decreased

9. Junctional pacemakers are _____ dependable. | not

10. Another danger is that faster, irritable ectopic foci may _____ _____ as pacemaker. | take over

11. Junctional rhythm may be a _____ of more serious arrhythmias. | warning or forerunner

12. There (is/is no) specific drug therapy for slow junctional rhythm. | is no

13. Transvenous _____ may be used to increase the rate and the cardiac output. | pacing

14. Lidocaine usually (is/is not) effective in suppressing ectopic beats occurring with slow junctional rhythm. | is not

PAROXYSMAL JUNCTIONAL TACHYCARDIA
(*ICC, 4th ed., pp. 168-169*)

Exercise 5

1. The pacemaker is the _____ _____. | junctional tissue

2. The rate is usually _____ to _____ beats per minute. | 140, 220

3. Possible causes of PJT are _____ imbalances and (increased/decreased) catecholamine secretions. | metabolic, increased

4. PJT may also be caused by _____ of the AV nodal area. — ischemia

5. An overdose of _____ may also cause it. — digitalis

6. PJT usually starts and stops _____ or _____. — abruptly, paroxysmally

7. The rapid ventricular rate can lead to _____ _____ _____. — left ventricular failure

8. If the rapid rate persists, the patient would probably (be/not be) comfortable. — not be

9. PJT (is/is not) considered dangerous. — is

10. If PJT cannot be differentiated from PAT, you may call it _____ _____ _____ _____. — paroxysmal supraventricular tachycardia (PSVT)

11. List some of the complications that may be produced by sustained PJT. _____ _____. — left ventricular failure, angina, cerebral ischemia

12. Initial treatment of PJT is _____ _____. — vagal stimulation

13. One way is by _____ _____ _____. — carotid sinus massage

14. If symptoms develop, PJT should be terminated promptly with _____ _____ _____. — synchronized precordial shock

15. If digitalis toxicity is suspected as a cause, the drug should be _____. — withheld

16. If your patient is not over-digitalized and is comfortable, IV _____ or _____ may be tried. — digitalis propranolol

17. Therapy to prevent recurrent episodes might include the drugs _____, _____, or _____. — propranolol, quinidine, digitalis

NONPAROXYSMAL JUNCTIONAL TACHYCARDIA
(*ICC, 4th ed., pp. 170-172*)

Exercise 6

1. The inherent pacing rate of junctional tissue is _____ to _____ beats per minute. — 40, 60

2. If the junctional area initiates impulses faster than 40 to 60 beats per minute, you could term it a _____ for the junctional cells. — tachycardia

3. The rates in nonparoxysmal tachycardia are between _____ and _____ beats per minute. — 70, 130

4. A more appropriate name might be _____ _____ rhythm (AJR). — accelerated junctional

5. AJR often is associated with _____ _____ _____ and _____ _____. — congestive heart failure cardiogenic shock

6. It can also be caused by what drug? _____ — digitalis

7. AJR often warns of further _____ displacement of the pacemaker. — downward

8. Symptoms are usually related to _____ _____ _____. — left ventricular failure (or CHF)

9. There (is/is not) a specific treatment for AJR. — is not

10. _____ _____ may be used because of the danger of downward displacement of the pacemaker. — Transvenous pacing

PUTTING IT TOGETHER (*ICC, 4th ed., Chapter 11*)
Exercise 7

Okay, back to your make-believe CCU. You've identified a change in a patient's monitor pattern. The P waves are inverted and the PR intervals are short. The QRS is normal.

132

1. To begin with, you should decide if the monitor is showing a _____ rhythm.

junctional

2. Now consider the rate. If the rate is between 40 and 60, you probably are seeing _____ _____.

junctional rhythm

3. If the rate is between 70-130, the patient is likely to have _____.

AJR

4. A rate of 140-220 would indicate a _____.

PJT

5. If the QRS is normal and the rate isn't too bad, you do not need to bother the doctor at night about this. (True/False)

False. You'd better!

6. Junctional rhythm and tachycardias (are/are not) considered warnings of impending danger.

are

7. If the patient's dose of digitalis is due, you'd want to _____ _____.

consult the doctor before giving it

8. If the junctional rhythm is slow, you could anticipate that the doctor might want to _____.

insert a transvenous pacemaker

12

Arrhythmias Originating in the Ventricles

When the pacemaker of an ischemic heart has retreated to the ventricles, there's not much room for further downward displacement. This is it; the bottom of the totem pole. And while infrequent, single focus (unifocal) PVCs may not be dangerous, they certainly keep nurses alert! Let's learn when to chew our finger nails and when to defibrillate.

VENTRICULAR ARRHYTHMIAS
(*ICC, 4th ed., p. 177*)

Exercise 1

1. An arrhythmia originating above the ventricles is called _____.

   supraventricular

2. Ventricular arrhythmias start below the _____ _____ _____.

   AV nodal area

3. Normal people may have PVCs that cause no problem. (True/False)

   True

4. PVCs are dangerous for the patient who has had an _____.

   MI

5. The progression of dangerous arrhythmias is:
   premature _____ contractions →
   ventricular _____ →
   Ventricular _____

   ventricular
   tachycardia
   fibrillation

6. The rate of ventricular tachycardia is _____ to _____ per minute.

   140, 250

7. Ventricular tachycardia is really a series of _____.

   PVCs

8. If you see on the monitor a rhythm that looks like ventricular tachycardia with a rate of 50 to 100/minute, you'd call it _____ _____ rhythm.

   accelerated idioventricular

9. This ventricular arrhythmia (does/does not) lead to ventricular fibrillation.

   does not

10. Ventricular tachycardia (does/does not) lead to ventricular fibrillation.

    does

135

11. So if you see what appears to be a continual string of PVCs you should _____ _____.	count the rate
12. 'Ratewise' (under/over) 100 is not so dangerous; (under/over) 140 is dangerous.	under, over

PREMATURE VENTRICULAR CONTRACTIONS
(ICC, 4th ed., pp. 178-180)

For a long time I've been promising that we would learn more about PVCs and ventricular fibrillation. The time has come. Pin on your hat and let's go.

Exercise 2

1. A contraction occurring before the regularly expected sinus beat is _____.	premature
2. A PVC is a premature contraction originating from an irritable focus in the _____.	ventricle
3. The most common ventricular arrhythmia is the _____.	PVC
4. The most common of *all* arrhythmias is the _____.	PVC
5. In PVCs the QRS will be (wide/narrow).	wide
6. A wide QRS measures more than _____ second.	0.12
7. The QRS will be (normal/abnormal) in shape.	abnormal
8. The abnormal QRS is described as _____ in shape.	distorted
9. The T wave usually (is/is not) the opposite direction from the QRS of the PVC.	is
10. Thus, if the PVC had a negative (downward) QRS, the T wave probably would be _____.	positive (upright)
11. If the PVC has a positive (upright) QRS, the T wave probably would be _____ _____. (*Note*: Questions 10 and 11 are "probably," not absolutely.)	nega- tive (downward)
12. Measuring from the normal QRS before the PVC to the normal QRS after the PVC should equal _____ R-R intervals.	2
13. This delay after a PVC is called a full _____ _____.	compensatory pause
14. In summary: PVCs can be diagnosed by a QRS that is _____ in shape and over _____ wide.	distorted 0.12 seconds
15. The T wave is probably in the _____ direction from the QRS,	opposite
16. and there should be a full _____ _____.	compensatory pause

If you work with monitored patients, you'll see PVCs every day, and you must be able to recognize them. You'll use the criteria we just reviewed to determine when you're seeing a PVC. Never forget these criteria!

DANGEROUS PVCs *(ICC, 4th ed., pp. 181-183)*

Now that we can recognize PVCs, we need to know when to intelligently fear them. The figures on pages 181-183 of *ICC*, 4th ed. are beautiful guides for recognizing different types of PVCs. Study these pages carefully. If you can't diagnose PVCs, you'll be miserable as a CCU nurse.

Exercise 3

1. PVCs usually indicate ventricular _____.	irritability
2. They may also be caused by drugs, especially _____.	digitalis

3. Patients with a low level of the electrolyte _____ tend to develop PVCs.	potassium
4. Potassium may be depleted during _____ therapy.	diuretic
5. Low potassium is called _____.	hypokalemia
6. Isolated, infrequent PVCs usually (are/are not) dangerous.	are not
7. Increasing numbers of PVCs indicate (increasing/decreasing) irritability.	increasing
8. Increased ventricular irritability can lead to ventricular _____.	tachycardia
9. Ventricular tachycardia can progress to ventricular _____.	fibrillation
10. You know how many PVCs per minute your patient has because you _____ them on the monitor. Which is more dangerous, 2 PVCs per minute or 7 per minute?	count (document) 7
11. If you see _____ or more PVCs a minute, you'd consider them very dangerous.	6 (some doctors say 5 per minute)
12. If every other beat is a PVC, the rhythm is called _____.	bigeminy
13. Ventricular bigeminy (is/is not) dangerous.	is
14. A PVC falling on the _____ wave of the preceding QRS is particularly dangerous.	T
15. This is called an _____-_____-_____ pattern.	R-on-T
16. PVCs originating from more than one ectopic focus are called _____.	multifocal
17. How do you know they come from more than one focus? _____ _____ _____	Because of the differences in the configuration of the PVC
18. Multifocal PVCs are usually (more/less) dangerous than unifocal PVCs.	more
19. _____ consecutive PVCs, known as couplets or_____, are especially dangerous.	Two, pairs
20. In summary, the dangerous PVCs are:	
A. _____ or more per minute,	6
B. _____ (every other beat)	bigeminal
C. _____-_____-_____ pattern,	R-on-T
D. _____ focal, and	multi
E. _____ in a row.	two

TREATMENT OF PVCs (ICC, 4th ed., p. 180)

Now that we can recognize PVCs and know when they're dangerous, what do we do about them?

Exercise 4

1. The primary drug treatment for PVCs is _____.	lidocaine
2. A trade name for lidocaine is _____.	Xylocaine
3. Initially, lidocaine is given as a _____ dose, IV.	push or bolus
4. The usual push dosage is _____ to _____ mg.	50, 100
5. Lidocaine should then be continued as an IV _____.	drip
6. An overdose of lidocaine can cause _____.	convulsions
7. If lidocaine fails, _____ can be tried.	procainamide

137

8. Procainamide and Pronestyl (are/are not) the same.

are

9. Pronestyl may cause the blood pressure to (drop/rise).

drop

10. Antiarrhythmic drugs sometimes used to control PVCs are _____ and _____.

'quinidine
dispyramide

11. Oral agents (should/should not) be used for emergency treatment of PVCs.

should not

12. Potassium (can/cannot) be used to suppress PVCs.

can

One rule of thumb about treating PVCs: the lidocaine drip should usually not be administered faster than 4 mg per minute. Respect lidocaine: the convulsions brought on by an overdose are unbelievable. Respect Pronestyl: your patient's blood pressure can "fall through the floor" with it.

VENTRICULAR TACHYCARDIA
(*ICC, 4th ed., pp. 184-187*)

PVCs → ventricular tachycardia → ventricular fibrillation: a progression you'll do your best to stop. Though ventricular tachycardia is in the middle of the scale, it's definitely an acute emergency (and that's worse than a plain emergency). The ECGs on pages 185-187 of *ICC*, 4th ed., depict ventricular tachycardia beautifully. Study them and don't forget them!

Exercise 5

1. Ventricular tachycardia is defined as _____ or more PVCs in a row.

3 (some doctors say 4 or more)

2. It's caused by severe _____ irritability.

ventricular

3. Ventricular tachycardia is often an immediate forerunner of _____ _____.

ventricular
fibrillation

4. Ventricular tachycardia (may/may not) occur in short runs or bursts.

may

5. It may stop spontaneously after a few seconds. (True/False)

True

6. But this would be a rare event. (True/False)

False

7. With sustained ventricular tachycardia, cardiac output is likely to _____.

fall

8. Decreased cardiac output may lead to _____ _____ failure.

left ventricular

9. Or worse, it may lead to _____ _____.

cardiogenic shock

10. Ventricular tachycardia can suddenly change to _____ _____.

ventricular
fibrillation

11. All of this means that ventricular tachycardia is an extremely _____ arrhythmia.

dangerous

Exercise 6

1. If ventricular tachycardia stops abruptly, you can sit back and forget about it. (True/False)

False

2. There is a (low/high) risk of further episodes.

high

3. Why? _____

The underlying problem is still present

4. Therefore treatment is necessary to prevent _____ _____.

further attacks

5. Ventricular tachycardia (often abbreviated to "V. Tach") is treated with _____.

lidocaine

138

6. The initial treatment is a push dose containing _____ mg.   100

7. After the push dose, continue lidocaine in an _____ _____.   IV drip

8. Some doctors use _____ _____ if lidocaine fails.   bretylium tosylate

9. If V. Tach continues despite the push dose of lidocaine, the next step is_____ _____.   precordial shock

10. Repeated attacks of this arrhythmia may be due to an electrolyte imbalance called _____.   hypokalemia

11. This means low _____.   potassium

12. It would be wise to have the _____ at the bedside once a patient has had V. Tach.   defibrillator

13. _____ _____ could develop very suddenly.   Ventricular defibrillation

MONITOR PRACTICE (PVCs AND VENTRICULAR TACHYCARDIA (*ICC, 4th ed., pp. 178-187*)

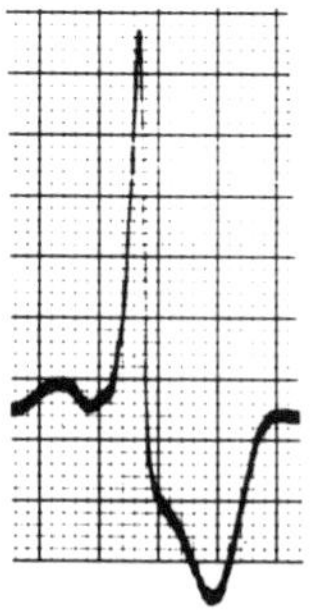

PVCs

**The bigger they are
The faster Nurse runs,
More dangerous by far:
Multifocal wee ones.**

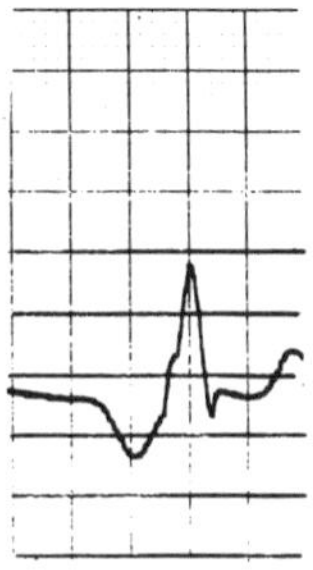

Figure 12.1.   **Figure 12.2.**

Exercise 7

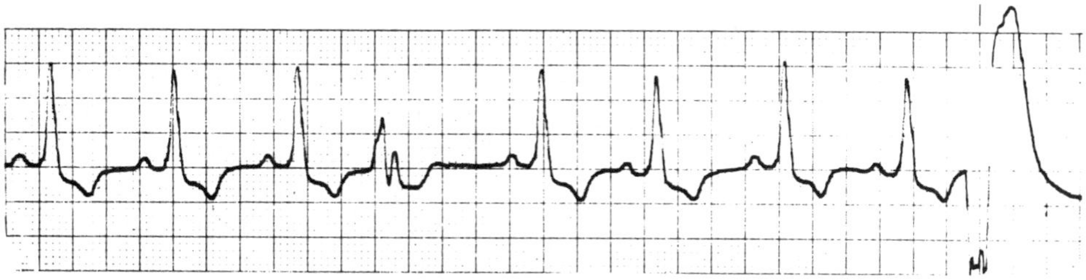

Figure 12.3. MR. P.B.

1. In 6 seconds our patient has had _____ PVCs.   2

2. Assuming he continues at this rate, he'll have _____ PVCs per minute.   20

3. You treat PVCs when they're over _____ per minute so give him a bolus of _____—fast!   6
lidocaine

4. How many foci of PVCs do you see? _____   2

5. Multifocal PVCs are _____ dangerous than unifocal. It shouldn't surprise you too much that this irritable heart went into ventricular tachycardia in the middle of the night. (He responded to lidocaine, recovered, and eventually went home.)   more

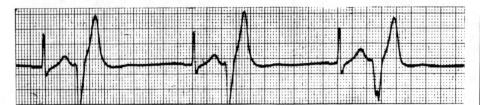

Figure 12.4. MR. B. JIMMINY.

6. Every other beat is a _____ _____
   _____ .

premature ventricular contraction

7. This is called _____ .

bigeminy

8. The PVCs are (unifocal/multifocal).

unifocal (they all have the same configuration)

9. When do the PVCs strike in relation to the T waves? _____
   _____

right after the T wave

10. Bigeminy might lead to _____
    _____ .

ventricular tachycardia or ventricular fibrillation

11. You'd treat these ectopic beats with _____ .

lidocaine

12. Sometimes bigeminy is a sign of _____ toxicity.

digitalis

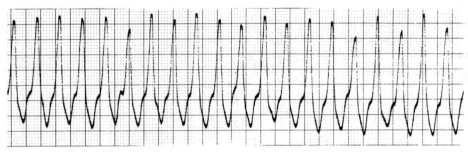

Figure 12.5. MR. V. T.

13. PVCs all in a row and at a rate of _____
    per minute!

200 (20 PVCs in 6 seconds)

14. Run, don't walk, with a syringe of _____ .

lidocaine

15. At any moment Mr. V.T. might develop _____ .

ventricular fibrillation

16. Bring the _____ to the bedside.

defibrillator

The alarm sounds and you see the ECG in Figure 12.6.

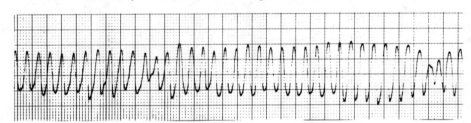

Figure 12.6. MS. O. LORD.

17. The diagnosis of _____
    seems likely, but you can't be sure.

ventricular flutter (very rapid ventricular tachycardia)

18. The first thing you'd do is _____ the patient.

examine

19. You must find out if she's _____ ____ _____ .

conscious or unconscious

20. She complains of marked shortness of breath. No wonder, her ventricular rate is
    nearly _____ !

400 per minute

21. You'd inject _____ instantly. lidocaine

22. It doesn't work. What now? You'd _____ the patient without delay. defibrillate

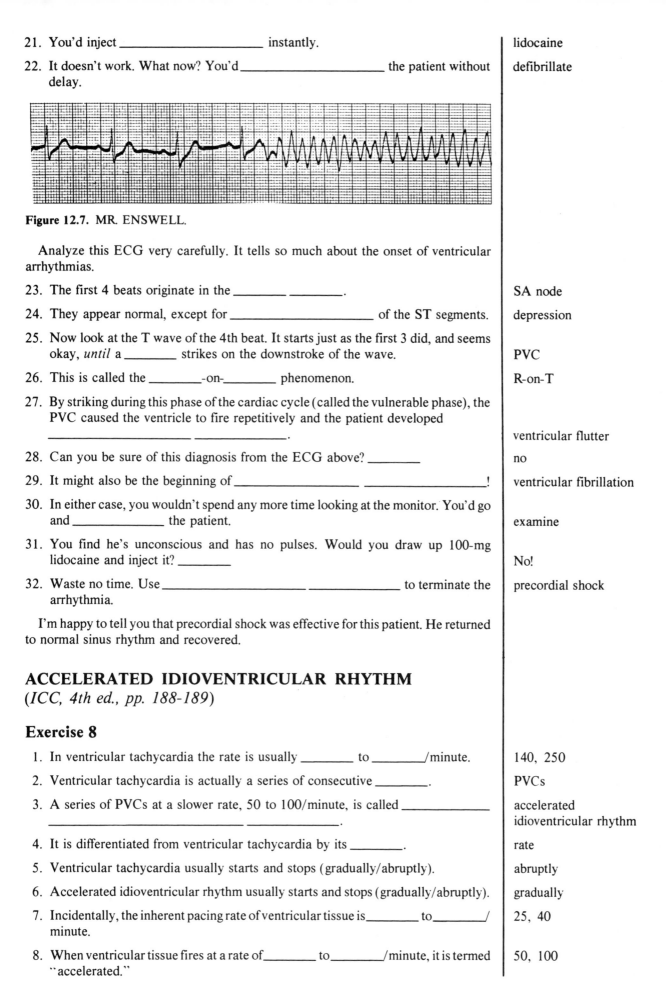

Figure 12.7. MR. ENSWELL.

Analyze this ECG very carefully. It tells so much about the onset of ventricular arrhythmias.

23. The first 4 beats originate in the _____ _____. SA node

24. They appear normal, except for _____ of the ST segments. depression

25. Now look at the T wave of the 4th beat. It starts just as the first 3 did, and seems okay, *until* a _____ strikes on the downstroke of the wave. PVC

26. This is called the _____-on-_____ phenomenon. R-on-T

27. By striking during this phase of the cardiac cycle (called the vulnerable phase), the PVC caused the ventricle to fire repetitively and the patient developed _____ _____. ventricular flutter

28. Can you be sure of this diagnosis from the ECG above? _____ no

29. It might also be the beginning of _____ _____! ventricular fibrillation

30. In either case, you wouldn't spend any more time looking at the monitor. You'd go and _____ the patient. examine

31. You find he's unconscious and has no pulses. Would you draw up 100-mg lidocaine and inject it? _____ No!

32. Waste no time. Use _____ _____ to terminate the arrhythmia. precordial shock

I'm happy to tell you that precordial shock was effective for this patient. He returned to normal sinus rhythm and recovered.

ACCELERATED IDIOVENTRICULAR RHYTHM
(*ICC, 4th ed., pp. 188-189*)

Exercise 8

1. In ventricular tachycardia the rate is usually _____ to _____/minute. 140, 250

2. Ventricular tachycardia is actually a series of consecutive _____. PVCs

3. A series of PVCs at a slower rate, 50 to 100/minute, is called _____ _____ _____. accelerated idioventricular rhythm

4. It is differentiated from ventricular tachycardia by its _____. rate

5. Ventricular tachycardia usually starts and stops (gradually/abruptly). abruptly

6. Accelerated idioventricular rhythm usually starts and stops (gradually/abruptly). gradually

7. Incidentally, the inherent pacing rate of ventricular tissue is _____ to _____/minute. 25, 40

8. When ventricular tissue fires at a rate of _____ to _____/minute, it is termed "accelerated." 50, 100

141

9. If the _____ nodal rate slows due to _____ or _____ toxicity, an accelerated ventricular pacemaker can take over.

SA, ischemia, digitalis

10. This (is/is not) a dangerous arrhythmia.

is not

11. Its only danger would be if it occurs together with ventricular _____.

tachycardia

12. The drug, _____, may be used to increase the SA nodal rate.

atropine

13. If the patient is receiving regular doses of _____, you'd call the doctor before giving the next dose.

digitalis

VENTRICULAR FIBRILLATION (*ICC, 4th ed., pp. 190-191*)

This ECG pattern is one of the most awesome you'll ever see: Ventricular Fibrillation!

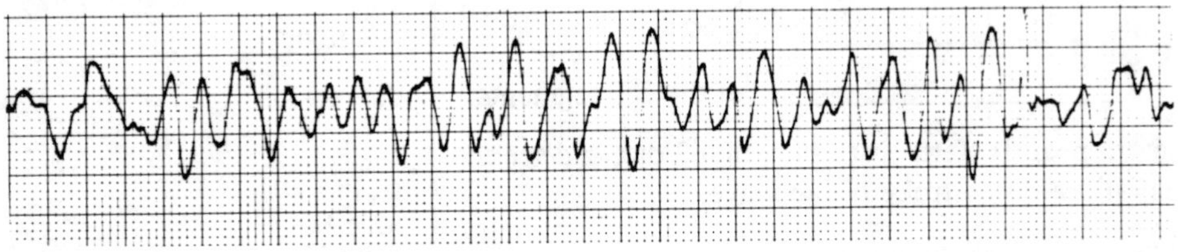

Figure 12.8.

Exercise 9

1. In ventricular fibrillation the heart muscles merely _____.

twitch

2. The ventricles (do/do not) contract.

do not

3. The ventricles (do/do not) pump blood.

do not

4. Would you find any pulse in a patient with ventricular fibrillation? _____

no

5. How would this patient appear? _____ or _____.

unconscious, convulsing

6. Ventricular fibrillation is probably caused by chaotic _____ activity in the ventricle.

electrical

7. It is generally preceded by _____.

PVCs

8. It (can/cannot) develop in a patient who is doing well clinically.

can

9. This is called _____ ventricular fibrillation.

primary

10. Primary ventricular fibrillation (can/cannot) be successfully defibrillated in most instances.

can

11. When ventricular fibrillation develops in patients with advanced left ventricular failure, it is called _____ ventricular fibrillation.

secondary

12. Secondary ventricular fibrillation (seldom/usually) can be defibrillated.

seldom

13. The average time between the onset of ventricular fibrillation and death is about _____.

2 minutes

14. This means defibrillation must be accomplished within _____.

2 minutes

Okay, keep the above information in mind, and let's imagine that we are at the bedside of the patient whose monitor pattern shows ventricular fibrillation.

Exercise 10

1. Rule number one: Always treat the _____, not the monitor.

patient

2. Check the patient. If he has ventricular fibrillation, you'll find no peripheral _____.

pulses

142

3. You will hear no _____ _____ with a stethoscope. (And don't waste time running for a stethoscope if you haven't one hanging around your neck.) — heart sounds

4. You will find no _____ _____. (Again, I wouldn't waste time running for equipment; if other signs were positive, I wouldn't even waste time checking it.) — blood pressure

5. The patient will probably be _____. — unconscious

6. The pupils soon (dilate/constrict). — dilate

7. The patient's color probably is _____. — cyanotic

8. He (may/may not) convulse. — may

9. What should you do? _____ — Defibrillate him, STAT.

Think of that! You must reach the bedside, diagnose by checking the patient as well as the monitor, and defibrillate him—all within 2 minutes. (Come back here, you don't have time to run for help!) It *can* be done, but don't pat yourself on the back until you can do it in less than 2 minutes. You may have to make some changes in the physical set-up in your hospital to save time, and you'll have to run some practice drills. But it is possible, and it's a tremendous thrill to succeed—*you've saved someone's life!*

TREATMENT OF VENTRICULAR FIBRILLATION
(ICC, 4th ed., pp. 192-193)

Exercise 11

1. The first step is _____ or _____ of the problem. — recognition, diagnosis

2. The monitor tips you off, but you actually confirm the diagnosis at the _____. — bedside

3. You'll find that the patient is _____ and that he has no _____ _____. — unconscious / peripheral pulses

4. The only treatment for ventricular fibrillation is _____. — defibrillation

5. Defibrillation should be performed within _____ minutes or less. — 2

6. You should use the _____ energy setting for defibrillation. — maximum

7. These patients all develop acidosis called _____ _____. — lactic acidosis

8. Lactic acidosis can be treated with _____ _____ IV. — sodium bicarbonate

9. After successful defibrillation, you must prevent _____. — recurrences

10. The best prevention is continuous IV _____. — lidocaine

NURSING ROLE IN VENTRICULAR FIBRILLATION *(ICC, 4th ed., p. 193)*

Read page 193 of *ICC*, 4th ed., very, very carefully. You won't have time to read it when ventricular fibrillation strikes.

Exercise 12

Now see if you can recall the first nine steps of the nursing role. I'll start you off. (Don't go into details of the defibrillation process yet; we'll do that in the next exercise.)

1. Monitor alarm sounds

2.

3.

4.

5.

6.

7.

8.

9.

Check your answers with page 193 *ICC*, 4th ed., and repeat this exercise until you can list all nine steps. Picture yourself doing each step as you list it.

Exercise 13

Now concentrate on the process of defibrillation as you would perform it. After you complete these statements, check your answers with the discussion that follows.

1. Before turning the machine on, spread _____ on the paddles.

2. Turn the defibrillator _____.

3. Set energy level at _____.

4. And be sure synchronizer is _____.

5. Place paddles on the chest so the current will go _____ the heart.

6. Hold the paddles _____ on the chest.

7. When discharging the shock, do not lean against the _____.

8. Be sure no one else touches the _____.

9. And do not touch the _____,_____ yourself except through the paddles with insulated handles.

10. Let everybody know you're ready to deliver the shock by saying _____.

11. If you have successfully defibrillated the patient, the monitor should no longer show _____.

12. If you're successful, your patient's circulation returns: what three signs should you find? _____, _____, _____.

13. Suppose you don't succeed, and the monitor still shows ventricular fibrillation; you'd _____ again.

14. But after two or three unsuccessful shocks, you would stop, and start _____ STAT.

15. Patients with ventricular fibrillation will almost always develop _____ _____, and you'll need _____ _____ to treat it.

16. If your patient is still in ventricular fibrillation and you're doing effective CPR and have sodium bicarbonate running in, then try _____ again.

Answers and Discussion

1. *Electrode paste or jelly.* Rub the paddles together to evenly spread the paste. DO THIS WITH THE DEFIBRILLATOR TURNED OFF, PLEASE! Instead of the paste, some hospitals use saline-soaked gauze pads. Place the pads on the chest and press the defibrillator paddles firmly over them. The pads must be wet, but not dripping; a trickle of saline running across the chest can conduct a spark and possibly burn the skin. The advantage of saline pads is that they don't leave a lot of slippery goop on the chest to interfere with cardiopulmonary resuscitation, should it be needed.

144

2-3-4. Ready to go? Turn the defibrillator *ON*, set energy level at *MAXIMUM* (400 watt-seconds); synchronizer must be *OFF*.

5. *Across* the heart. Do not put the paddles on the monitor electrodes or wires—you may defibrillate the monitor. When attaching the monitor electrodes it's wise to initially leave open space on the chest for defibrillation; nobody has time to reposition monitor leads before defibrillating a patient.

6. *Firmly.* Don't rock or tip them. If you do, you may produce a fireworks display and burn the patient in the process. Worse, the current may not go through to the heart.

7-8-9. Three safety rules: nobody touches the *patient*, or the *bed*, or the *defibrillator cart.* Don't lean over and touch any of these yourself. If you are delivering the shock, it's up to you to insure everyone else's safety. And if you work with some knuckleheaded doctor who insists he's going to continue with CPR or "bagging" (breathing) the patient while you shock, tell him that he must move away or you may have to defibrillate him, too.

10. Even if you must shout, be sure everyone knows when you're going to defibrillate. I don't care if you say, *"Fire!" "Shock!" "Ready—go!"* Say something!

11. *Fibrillation.* Sometimes the pattern after defibrillation isn't exactly normal, but if ventricular fibrillation has stopped and the patient's condition improves, don't defibrillate again; just hang in there.

12. The patient's *pulses* return; he has a measurable *blood pressure*; his *color* improves, *pupils constrict*, and, the greatest joy of all, he says, "Hey, watcha' do that for?"

13. *Defibrillate.*

14. *CPR*—before there's any chance of brain damage. How long have you spent defibrillating? Five minutes? Too long. Two minutes? That's more like it. Do CPR for a few minutes to circulate blood and oxygen to the brain, then defibrillate again if fibrillation continues. Remember, fibrillation does NOT circulate the blood; you must do that with CPR.

15. *Lactic acidosis* will occur; get the *sodium bicarbonate* going. One hint: if you must draw up sodium bicarbonate into a syringe, get the largest needle you can find. It may look clear in the vial, but it's as thick as pea soup when you try to draw it up.

16. *Defibrillation.* If you're circulating oxygen to the brain and counteracting lactic acidosis and he's still fibrillating—shock him again. Sometimes intracardiac or IV epinephrine is given to "strengthen" the fibrillation, and then defibrillation may be successful. With more than one nurse present, these things can be done almost simultaneously. Just don't shock your CPR givers and your IV helper—you need them!

Exercise 14

He's been in the CCU for 2 days and hasn't had any serious complications. Suddenly the alarm rings! You look at the monitor and see this:

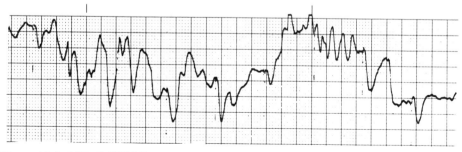

Figure 12.9. MR. B. WARE.

No question about it—ventricular fibrillation. You grab the defibrillator and race to the bedside, not a second lost. You slop the electrode paste on and—STOP! Mr. Ware opens his eyes and protests, "Hey, what are ya doin'? What's goin' on?"

1. Mr. Ware (is/is not) in ventricular fibrillation.

is not

2. The electrical pattern is probably an _____.

artifact

3. The point is: always treat the _____ and not the _____!

patient, monitor

Although the ECG looks like ventricular fibrillation, Mr. Ware would certainly *not* be alert and talking to you if this really were the problem. We are seeing an *artifact* on the monitor: Something has happened to the electrodes or the machine. Remember: treat the *patient*, not the *monitor*.

13

Disorders of Conduction

CLASSIFICATION OF CONDUCTION DISORDERS
(*ICC, 4th ed., pp. 199-201*)

Exercise 1

One of the basic premises of medicine is that nearly everything has three names. The classification of conduction disorders is no exception. So hang in there, and let's see how you do.

1. A conduction disorder implies that the impulse originates _____, but that its conduction is _____ at some point thereafter.

    normally (in the SA node)
    blocked

2. Initially, the impulse can be blocked before it ever leaves the_____ _____.

    SA node

3. Or the impulse can make it into the atria where it can be blocked in the_____ tracts.

    internodal

4. These disorders would be classified as blocks in the _____ node.

    SA

5. Incidentally, you cannot differentiate these blocks from _____ _____ on an ECG.

    SA arrest

6. If an impulse that originated in the SA node makes it through the atria, it could be blocked in the _____ node, or in the area surrounding the node, called the _____ area.

    AV
    junctional

7. Because this area of blockage is between the atria and ventricles, we can call it an _____ block.

    atrioventricular

8. This area is a junction, or joining area, so we can substitute the phrase "_____ block."

    junctional

9. If the electrical impulse makes it through the junctional area, it has successfully passed *through* the _____ _____ _____ to its bifurcation.

    bundle of His

10. The impulse can still be blocked below the level of_____ of the bundle of His.

    bifurcation

11. Blocks below the bifurcation, because they are within the ventricles, can be termed _____ blocks.

    intraventricular

12. Or, because they are below the junctional area, they are sometimes called _____ blocks.

    subjunctional

147

Exercise 2

This all may seem a little complicated, so let's try it in diagrammatic fashion. Label the following picture to see if you can visualize the areas where conduction blocks occur.

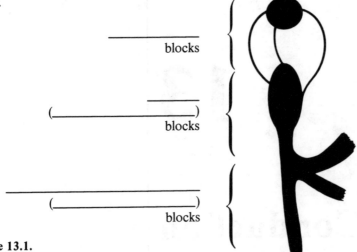

_____ blocks

(_____)
blocks

_____
(_____)
blocks

Figure 13.1.

SA node
blocks

AV
(junctional)
blocks

Intraventricular
(subjunctional)
blocks

ATRIOVENTRICULAR BLOCKS

We'll skip over SA node and atrial blocks because they really can't be differentiated from sinus arrest. In any event they are treated in the same fashion.

Atrioventricular (or junctional) blocks are divided into three classes. To picture them clearly, we need to use our imaginations. Suppose we think of the heart as being a very old-fashioned (no elevator), but very fancy, two-story apartment house. Access to the stairway between floors is controlled by a doorman, tottery old Mr. A. V. Node. The upper floor is called The Atria and the lower floor is called The Ventricles. People (electrical impulses) must go down on a stairway to pass from The Atria to The Ventricles.

If Mr. A. V. Node is doing his job of opening the door properly as soon as an impulse arrives, it takes less than 0.20 seconds to travel from Atria to Ventricles. But A. V. Node sometimes slows down, and then it takes longer than 0.20 seconds for impulses to reach the Ventricles (first degree heart block). At other times he takes a rest and won't open the door for each impulse that arrives. He may block every second or third or fourth impulse from reaching the Ventricles (second degree heart block). Worst of all, A. V. Node may tire out and fall asleep. No impulses can then pass the nodal staircase—*all* are blocked (third degree heart block).

Exercise 3

Keeping old Mr. A. V. Node in mind, try the following questions to see if you have the basic ideas.

1. First, second, and third degree AV blocks are subdivisions of _____
   (or _____) blocks.

2. In 1st degree AV block the impulse is _____, but it is eventually _____ to the ventricles.

3. In 2nd degree AV block _____, but not _____, impulses are _____.

4. In 3rd degree AV block _____ impulses are _____.

5. Thus, _____ impulses are conducted from atria to ventricles in 3rd degree block.

atrioventricular
junctional

delayed
conducted

some, all, blocked

all, blocked

no

INTRAVENTRICULAR (SUBJUNCTIONAL) BLOCKS

Say goodbye to Mr. A. V. Node because we're leaving his territory. Now we're going to consider blocks occurring *below* the level of bifurcation of the bundle of His.

Exercise 4

1. Do you know what bifurcation means? If not, look it up.

   ??
   !!

2. Intraventricular blocks developing *after* an MI usually mean that there is_____ to the conduction pathways, probably in the interventricular_____ area.

   injury
   septal

3. Intraventricular blocks existing *before* an MI usually indicate a chronic _____ of the bundle branches.

   degeneration or scarring

Exercise 5

Ready to work on the anatomy and physiology of the bundle branches?

1. Electrical conduction passes through the AV node to the_____ _____ _____.

   bundle of
   His

2. The bundle of His divides into 2 main branches. One of those branches is called the *right bundle branch* or _____. (initials)

   RBB

3. The other branch is abbreviated as _____.

   LBB

4. The LBB divides almost immediately into 2 branches. Another term for branches is _____.

   fascicles

5. The fascicle serving the front portion of the heart would be called the _____ fascicle of the LBB.

   anterior

6. The branch going to the back of the heart would be called the _____ _____ of the LBB.

   posterior
   fascicle

7. Thus, there is a total of _____ fascicles.

   3 (2 from LBB, 1 from RBB)

So far, so good. Now let's consider where blocks could occur in the bundle branches. Use the initials for your answers.

8. A block in the main right bundle branch is called an _____.

   RBBB

9. A block in the main left bundle branch is called an _____.

   LBBB

10. A block in the anterior fascicle of the LBB is called an _____.

   LAH

11. The H in LAH stands for _____.

   hemiblock

12. A block in the posterior fascicle of the LBB is called an _____.

   LPH

13. Now suppose there's a block of the RBB plus one of the two left fascicles, you'd call it a _____ _____.

   bifascicular block (that's 2 of the 3 branches)

14. Or (really bad) a block of all three branches below the bundle of His would be a _____ _____.

   trifascicular block (all 3 branches)

Exercise 6

If you're having trouble with any of the material on conduction blocks, or if you just want to make sure you know it, try the Mix and Match below and on the next page. Write the correct mixers in front of the matches.

MIXERS	MATCHES	
1. SA block	_____ block in right bundle branch	5
2. 1st degree block	_____ block in anterior fascicle of left bundle branch	7
3. 2nd degree block	_____ AV node blocks *some* impulses	3
4. 3rd degree block	_____ block in SA node or atria	1
5. RBBB	_____ block in posterior fascicle of left bundle branch	8

6. LBBB	_____ AV node blocks all impulses	4
7. LAH	_____ block in all 3 bundle branch fascicles	10
8. LPH	_____ delay in conduction to ventricles	2
9. bisfascicular block	_____ block in left main bundle branch	6
10. trifascicular block	_____ block in the right bundle branch plus one fascicle of left bundle branch	9

FIRST DEGREE AV HEART BLOCK
(ICC, 4th ed., pp. 202-203)

Exercise 7

We haven't tried any true or false questions for a while, so let's try some. Note whether the statements below are true or false. Remember, they all refer to first-degree AV block.

_____	1. Does not reduce hemodynamic efficiency of the heart.	T
_____	2. Delayed conduction shows in the PR interval.	T
_____	3. Vagal overactivity can be a cause.	T
_____	4. Does affect rate or rhythm.	F
_____	5. PR interval longer than 0.28 is more dangerous.	T
_____	6. PR interval is 0.21 or greater.	T
_____	7. Usually treat only if it's progressive or extreme.	T
_____	8. Atropine is not a treatment.	F
_____	9. Antiarrhythmic drugs can be a cause.	T
_____	10. Impulses are blocked in the AV node.	F
_____	11. Diagnosis is by ECG.	T
_____	12. Atropine 0.1 to 0.5 mg IV is standard treatment.	F
_____	13. Prepare for transvenous pacing if progressive.	T
_____	14. Notify doctor if PR is greater than 0.28.	T
_____	15. Digitalis is not a possible cause.	F
_____	16. Caused by ischemia of the AV node.	T
_____	17. Patient is aware of sensation of irregularity.	F
_____	18. May warn of impending second or third degree block.	T
_____	19. Is a serious arrhythmia in its own right.	F
_____	20. Don't begin treatment unless PR is 0.36 or greater.	F

SECOND DEGREE AV BLOCK—WENCKEBACH
(TYPE I) *(ICC, 4th ed., pp. 204-206)*

Exercise 8

Second degree heart block—this is where our doorman, AV Node, blocks some but not all conduction between the atria and ventricles. Sometimes the old gentleman tries hard to keep up with his job. However, he tires out and takes longer to allow each impulse through the conduction stairway. Finally, he has to take a brief rest and, as a result, one impulse is blocked from reaching the ventricles. He then feels refreshed and goes back to work, starting the cycle all over again. How do we know this about AV Node's behavior? The ECG shows us a series of increasingly prolonged PR intervals until one P wave is not followed by a QRS. After the blocked beat, the pattern repeats itself.

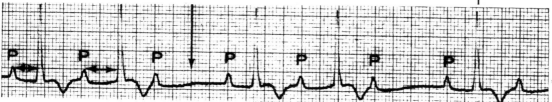

Figure 13.2. This conduction disturbance is called Wenckebach (wink-key-bok) type second degree block.

1. In Wenckebach blocks you'll find (more/fewer) P waves than QRSs.	more
2. The PR interval will (increase/decrease) with each beat.	increase
3. Finally, an impulse (is/is not) conducted.	is not
4. The ventricular rhythm (will/will not) be regular.	will not
5. The basic pacemaker is the _____ _____.	SA node
6. The problem lies in the _____ _____.	AV node
7. There is a (progressive/constant) slowing of conduction through the AV node.	progressive
8. This is the (mildest/severest) form of second degree heart block.	mildest
9. Wenckebach (can/cannot) progress to third degree block.	can
10. If the heart rate drops below 50, treatment with _____ is indicated.	isoproterenol

Exercise 9: Second Degree AV Block (Constant PR Interval) Type 2 (Mobitz)

You've just learned that Wenckebach is a form of second degree block in which the PR interval varies. Now we're going to compare this to second degree block with a constant PR but with some missing (blocked) QRSs.

1. Wenckebach is caused by an injury to the _____ _____.	AV node
2. In Type 2 (Mobitz), the block is (below/above) the AV junction; this is termed a _____ block.	below subjunctional
3. The manual uses the term 2:1 type second degree block; however, the block can be _____ or _____ etc.	3:1, 4:1
4. It may occasionally be caused by overdosage of _____.	digitalis
5. There are (more/fewer) P waves than QRSs.	more
6. In 2:1 block there are _____ P waves for each QRS.	2
7. In 3:1 block there are _____ P waves for each QRS.	3
8. 3:1 block (is/is not) the same as third degree heart block.	is not

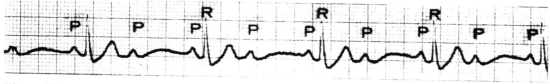

Figure 13.3.

Exercise 10

The following questions relate to second degree block with a constant PR.

1. The QRS complexes occur (regularly/irregularly) when the block is constant. | regularly

2. The P waves occur (regularly/irregularly). | regularly

3. The PR interval of the beats that are conducted (is/is not) constant. | is

4. The degree of block may change. (True/False) | True

5. Because the block is below the junction, a junctional pacemaker (can/cannot) take over. | cannot

6. Type 2 block is usually associated with (anterior/posterior) MIs. | anterior

7. The drug _____ is not a recommended treatment. | atropine

8. The more blocked beats, the more serious the block. (True/False) | True

9. 2:1 blocks (are/are not) stable. | are not

10. 2:1 blocks can be a forerunner of _____ _____ _____ or ventricular _____. | third degree block (complete) standstill

THIRD DEGREE HEART BLOCK
(ICC, 4th ed., pp. 210-213)

Exercise 11

In third degree block, old Mr. AV Node has had it. No impulses can reach the ventricle. The sinus impulses may continue to bombard the AV node regularly, but none of them is conducted to the ventricles. This is the condition we feared in patients with first and second degree heart block. This is what we had hoped to prevent. We now have a critical problem.

1. In third degree block the atria are paced by the _____ _____. | SA node

2. Thus, we see normal _____ waves. | P

3. (Some/All) of the P waves are blocked. | All

4. Another name for third degree block is _____ heart block. | complete

5. In acute MI, this block is usually caused by _____ damage of the junctional area. | ischemic

6. Since none of the atrial impulses reach the ventricles, what causes the ventricles to contract? _____ _____ | (Either a junctional or a ventricular pacemaker)

7. If the block occurs (above/below) the bifurcation of the bundle of _____, a junctional pacemaker may take over. | above, His

8. Junctional escape pacemakers can cause ventricular contraction at a rate of _____ to _____ per minute. | 40, 60

9. What will the atrial rate be? | Whatever the SA node is doing.

10. However, the block may occur *below* the _____ of the bundle of His, then the ventricular rate would probably be _____ to _____ per minute. | bifurcation 30, 40

11. The atrial rate will be (faster than/slower than/the same as) the ventricular rate, whether the block is above or below the bifurcation. | faster than

12. There (is/is not) a relationship between atrial and ventricular contractions. | is not

13. As a result, the PR interval (is/is not) constant. | is not

14. There (is/is not) a relationship between P waves and QRSs. | is not

152

15. You might say the atria and ventricles are divorced; the medical term for this is _____ _____.

    atrioventricular dissociation

16. The independent ventricular pacemaker (is/is not) dependable.

    is not

17. Effective contractions (may/may not) cease at any moment.

    may

18. This would cause a lethal arrhythmia: _____ _____.

    ventricular standstill

19. In addition, there is the threat of a faster ventricular focus taking over and causing _____.

    ventricular tachycardia or ventricular fibrillation

20. The ventricular rate (can/cannot) increase to meet circulatory demands.

    cannot

21. Thus the patient often has inadequate _____ _____.

    cardiac output

22. What cerebral symptoms might you expect in a patient with third degree heart block? _____, _____, _____, _____.

    confusion, lightheadedness fainting, convulsions

23. Syncopal episodes arising from decreased cerebral circulation are called _____-_____ attacks.

    Stokes-Adams

24. These patients may also develop symptoms of _____ _____ _____.

    left ventricular failure

25. Complete heart block (is/is not) an extremely dangerous arrhythmia.

    is

Exercise 12

Imagine you have just admitted a patient with complete heart block; treatment has not yet been started.

1. Your patient may suddenly _____ or _____.

   faint, convulse

2. The best overall treatment for complete heart block is _____ _____.

   transvenous pacing

3. Ideally, a transvenous pacing catheter should be inserted _____ third degree begins.

   before

4. A pacing catheter should be left in place at least _____ days after NSR is re-established.

   5

5. Unfortunately, in this patient, none is in place; therefore you should (get ready/wait for an order) for insertion of a pacing catheter.

   get ready

6. One drug that may help in the meantime is _____.

   Isuprel

7. There is a (good/poor) chance that complete heart block due to MI may subside in a few days.

   good

8. If third degree heart block does not subside, but becomes permanent, it can be treated with a permanent _____.

   pacemaker

Exercise 13

These questions also refer to the patient in complete heart block.

1. First, you must _____ or _____ the arrhythmia and document or record it.

   identify, diagnose

2. When would you call the doctor? _____

   STAT

3. What drug would you have ready? _____

   Isoproterenol

4. The order might be for _____ mg Isuprel in _____ cc dextrose in water IV.

   1, 250

5. You'd know that the drug should be given very _____.

   slowly

153

6. You'd watch the monitor for _____ _____.

7. This patient may suddenly go into ventricular _____.

8. So you'd bring the _____ to the bedside.

9. You'd also bring a syringe of 100 mg _____ or _____ to the bedside.

10. Where would you put the crash cart? _____

11. How does the patient feel about all this activity? _____

ectopic beats

fibrillation

defibrillator

lidocaine
xylocaine

at the bedside

scared!

Take a moment to consider this patient. He's terrified. Can you screen some of this awesome equipment, yet have it instantly ready? Can you be calm and matter-of-fact? Know where things are; know what you need. Be prepared. Then you can reassure this patient honestly and convincingly that everything possible is being done. Is it important to talk to this patient? Many patients describe a "fading away" and an enclosing blackness. They say the nurse's voice was their only reassurance.

I remember particularly a woman with third degree heart block whose transvenous pacemaker failed in the middle of the night. Her ventricular rate fell to about 35 per minute. And then she went into ventricular fibrillation. After we defibrillated her, she developed ventricular standstill. External pacing was only partially successful and she found it extremely painful. So we alternately used cardiopulmonary resuscitation, defibrillation and external pacing until the doctor arrived and inserted a new pacing catheter. Later, before she went home, she told us, "It was the sound of your voice that pulled me through. I'd climb up out of a dark pit and there'd be a horrible crushing on my chest. Then I'd hear a beautiful voice saying: 'Hang on, Mary, we won't let you die. Keep trying just a little bit longer.' And so I kept trying."

There are excellent examples of third degree heart block shown on pages 211-213 of the Manual. Measure out P-P and R-R intervals with your scrap paper. Prove to yourself that the atria and ventricles are divorced totally and completely. Measure the PR intervals and prove that they are never constant.

Exercise 14

Okay, let's set up our mythical CCU. You already have 3 patients and you're going to admit Mr. Percival Long and Mr. Adam Stokes. Let's check their monitors and answer some questions.

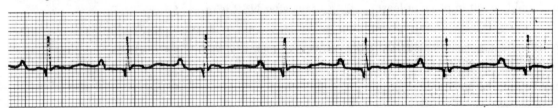

Figure 13.4. Mr. Percival Long.

This is an admission rhythm strip.

1. What is the ventricular rate? _____

70 per minute

2. Are the P waves normal? _____

yes

3. Are the QRS complexes normal? _____

yes

4. He is in _____ rhythm.

normal sinus

5. Then what's the problem? _____ _____ _____

The PR interval is prolonged to 0.28 seconds. This is first degree heart block.

6. What would you watch for in this patient? _____

signs of advancing heart block

7. Is any treatment necessary now? _____

no

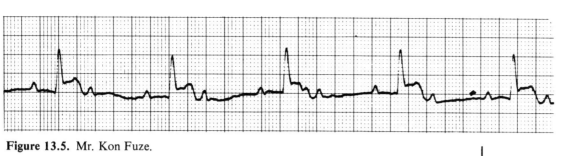

Figure 13.5. Mr. Kon Fuze.

Confused? Well let's see if we can make some sense out of this ECG.

1. Find the R waves. What is the ventricular rate? _____ | 50 per minute

2. Now pick out the P waves. Don't let that step-stool after the P waves fool you—it's an elevated _____ segment. | ST

3. How many P waves are there in this 6-second strip? _____ | 10

4. This means the atrial rate is _____ per minute. | 100 (10 × 10)

5. We now know the atrial rate is faster than the ventricular rate. There are_____ P waves for each _____ complex. | 2 QRS

6. This tells us that every other P wave is _____, and not conducted. | blocked

7. The PR interval of the conducted beats is (constant/inconstant). | constant

8. The PR interval of the conducted beats is _____ seconds. | 0.28

9. The interpretation of this ECG is _____ _____ heart block with _____ block. | second degree 2:1

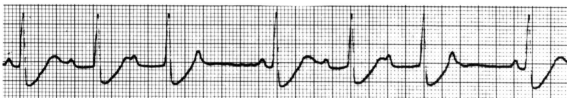

Figure 13.6. Mr. W. Bokman.

1. Is the rhythm regular? _____ | no

2. What is the ventricular rate? _____ | 70 per minute

3. Study the first 3 beats on the strip. What do you notice? _____ _____ | The PR interval increases with each beat

4. This means there is an increasing_____ in conduction through the AV node, | delay

5. until a beat is _____. | blocked

6. This is a form of_____ degree heart block. | second

7. It is called _____ type I block. | Wenckebach

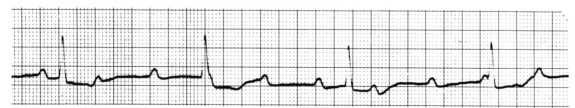

Figure 13.7. Ms. D. D.

She's in trouble, and we have to act quickly.

1. Her ventricular rate is only _____ per minute. | 40

155

2. Measure out her P waves. Use a scrap paper and mark the first three P waves, then keep moving the marks across the strip. Are the P waves regular? _____

    Yes, the P waves are regular

    Did you find the 4th and 9th P waves hidden in or near the QRS complexes?

3. What is the atrial rate? _____ per minute

    100 (10 P waves in 6 seconds × 10 = 100)

4. Is there any relationship between the P waves and QRS complexes? _____

    no

5. Are the PR intervals as constant as Mr. Kon Fuze's? _____
    _____

    No, the PR intervals are *not* constant

6. Ms. DD's atria and ventricles are divorced. She has developed _____
    _____

    third degree (complete) heart block

7. The slow ventricular rate is very dangerous because the cardiac output cannot be
    _____.

    maintained

8. There is also a threat of _____ _____ developing.

    ventricular fibrillation or ventricular standstill

9. What is the most dependable treatment for this problem? _____
    _____ _____.

    transvenous cardiac pacing

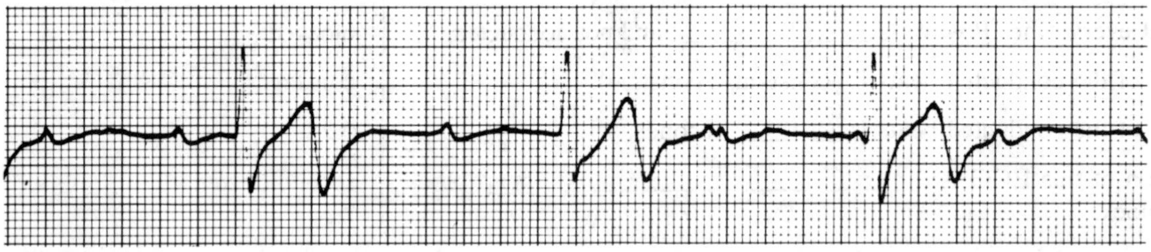

Figure 13.8. Mr. Adam Stokes.

This patient is unconscious when you admit him. You connect the monitor to this cold, clammy man and what do you see! (Can you imagine how you'd feel?)

1. The ventricular rate is just _____ per minute.

    30

2. The reason he's unconscious is that cerebral _____ is inadequate.

    blood flow (perfusion)

3. Are the atria beating faster than the ventricles? _____

    yes

4. Are the PR intervals constant? _____

    No

5. The ECG diagnosis is _____ _____ _____.

    complete heart block

6. As soon as you see this pattern, you'd _____,

    call the doctor stat

7. He's likely to order _____ IV until he gets there.

    isoproterenol (Isuprel)

8. While he's on his way, you'd prepare for _____ _____
    _____.

    transvenous cardiac pacing

INTRAVENTRICULAR (SUBJUNCTIONAL) BLOCKS
(*ICC, 4th ed., pp. 214-216*)

Are you sure of where we are? Just for orientation's sake, we're studying blocks *below* the AV junctional area, e.g., bundle branch blocks. Since bundle branch blocks imply that something is wrong with the conduction pathway, let's start with a brief review of electrical conduction through the heart and then move on to the BBB (bundle branch blocks).

Exercise 15

1. In first, second, or third degree blocks, the conduction disturbance is in or near the
    _____ _____.

    AV node

2. In bundle branch blocks (BBB), conduction is normal through the AV node. (True/False)

True

3. The problem arises below the _____ _____ _____.

bundle of His

4. The block is in either the _____ bundle branch or _____ bundle branch of the bundle of His.

left, right

5. This results in delayed activation of either the _____ or _____ ventricle, depending on which branch is blocked.

left, right

6. If the right bundle branch is blocked, the right ventricle is stimulated through the _____ _____.

interventricular septum

7. Consequently, the right ventricle would be stimulated (before/after) the left ventricle.

after

8. The time for both ventricles to be activated would be (longer/shorter) than normal.

longer

9. This delay is shown in the (PR/QRS) portion of the cycle.

QRS

10. The characteristic ECG finding of BBB is a prolonged _____ complex.

QRS

11. *Prolonged* means over _____ seconds in duration.

0.12

12. BBB may be (acute/chronic/both).

both

13. Chronic BBB is usually due to _____ of the bundle branches.

degeneration or scarring

14. Acute BBB develops as a complication of _____ _____.

acute MI

15. Acute BBB suggests that the _____ _____ has been injured.

interventricular septum

16. Prognosis in acute BBB is (better/worse) than in chronic BBB.

worse

Exercise 16

Use Figure 13.9 to help you understand the dangers of BBB.

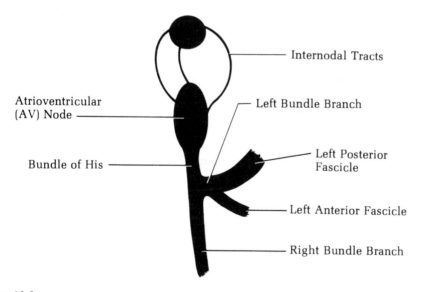

Figure 13.9.

1. An acute block of only one fascicle (is/is not) considered dangerous.

is

2. A block of the _____ bundle branch obscures the diagnosis of MI.

left

3. Blocks of _____ fascicles are more dangerous than blocks of one pathway.

2

4. If three pathways are blocked, _____ _____ may result.

ventricular standstill

157

5. Any degree of acute BBB indicates myocardial _____, especially of the _____ _____ area.

> damage
> interventricular septal

Exercise 17

Mr. M. I. has been in the CCU for two days. Except for occasional PVCs, no other arrhythmias have occurred. The QRS complexes have been 0.08 seconds. Today you notice that the QRS has widened to 0.14 seconds. The heart rate is 70 beats per minute and you can identify P waves before each QRS complex.

1. What is the most likely diagnosis? _____ _____

> A bundle branch block has developed

2. How do you know that the wide QRS complexes aren't PVCs? _____ _____

> P waves are seen before each complex

3. Can you tell from the monitor if this is an RBBB or LBBB? _____

> No

4. How can you make sure? _____

> Take a 12-lead ECG

5. Can you tell from the monitor how many fascicles are involved? _____

> No

6. How can you tell? _____

> With a 12-lead ECG

7. Should you call the doctor? _____

> Yes

8. Why? _____ _____

> Because this may be a warning of complete heart block or ventricular standstill

9. What treatment is likely to be used? _____ _____

> Insertion of transvenous pacemaker

10. Overdose of _____ might possibly cause BBB.

> quinidine

VENTRICULAR STANDSTILL (ICC, 4th ed., pp. 217-218)

Exercise 18

We've already discussed ventricular fibrillation. Now we come to the other sudden death arrhythmia—ventricular standstill (e.g., "Hey, look at the monitor. He's in asystole!"). Without a monitor, you can't tell the difference between the two sudden death arrhythmias. The circulation stops in both circumstances. And not so long ago, before we had coronary care units, the treatment was identical; at least we can save lives after ventricular fibrillation. But what about ventricular standstill? Well, the picture here isn't as bright. Most patients who develop ventricular standstill still die. But "most" doesn't mean *all*, and there's always a chance. With effective CPR we can maintain adequate circulation and hope that with pacing or drugs the doctor may be able to reverse this sudden death process.

1. There are two types of ventricular standstill, _____ and _____.

> primary, secondary

2. Primary ventricular standstill usually occurs without any previous ECG warning. (True/False)

> False

3. It usually develops in patients with _____ _____.

> heart block

4. Ventricular contractions _____ or become inadequate.

> cease

5. Inadequate cerebral circulation can cause _____.

> unconsciousness

6. Sometimes these attacks are transient and are called _____-_____ attacks.

> Stokes-Adams

7. During these attacks, cerebral circulation becomes inadequate and the patient loses _____.

> consciousness

8. Patients may survive Stokes-Adams attacks. (True/False)

> True

158

9. However, if ventricular standstill persists, it causes _____.	death
10. Primary ventricular standstill often can be prevented. (True/False)	True
11. Once it occurs, it can (possibly/almost never) be reversed.	possibly
12. If ventricular standstill develops in a patient with advanced circulatory failure, it is called _____ ventricular standstill.	secondary
13. In this situation, hypoxia and electrolyte imbalances depress the heart's _____ system.	electrical (or conduction)
14. The damage is usually reversible. (True/False)	False
15. Secondary ventricular standstill (sometimes/rarely) responds to CPR and cardiac pacing.	rarely
16. Which is more common, primary or secondary ventricular standstill?	secondary (unfortunately)
17. Another name for ventricular standstill is _____.	asystole

Exercise 19

The ECG pattern of ventricular standstill isn't as distinctive as ventricular fibrillation and may show itself in several different ways. Let's look at this rhythm strip and see if we can interpret what has happened.

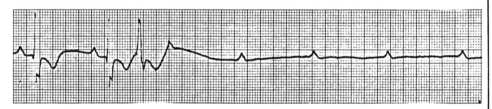

Figure 13.10.

1. The P waves of the first beats are normal and each is followed by a _____ complex.	QRS
2. This means the impulse was conducted from the atria to the _____.	ventricles
3. The third beat is an ectopic beat (probably a premature junctional contraction, but it doesn't really matter). It, too, has a _____ complex.	QRS
4. Suddenly, there are no more _____ complexes!	QRS
5. However, the _____ waves continue.	P
6. This means that the _____ are being stimulated, but the _____ aren't.	atria, ventricles
7. The absence of ventricular complexes indicates _____ _____.	ventricular standstill (or asystole)

Exercise 20

This patient had cardiogenic shock and was comatose when the following strip was taken.

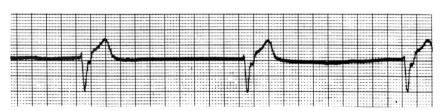

Figure 13.11.

159

1. Are P waves present? _____   no

2. This means the pacemaker is no longer in the _____ _____ or atria.   SA node

3. But it has descended to the _____ _____ or _____.   junctional area, ventricles

4. The ventricular complexes are _____ and _____.   wide, distorted

5. This electrical activity means the ventricles must be contracting normally. (True/False)   False

6. There is no blood pressure or pulse because the ventricles are not _____.   contracting

7. The electrical stimulus is _____ for ventricular contraction.   inadequate

8. The patient died minutes later. The ECG diagnosis: _____ _____ _____.   secondary ventricular standsill

9. Would pacing have helped this patient? _____   No, the heart couldn't respond

TREATMENT OF VENTRICULAR STANDSTILL
(*ICC, 4th ed., p. 219*)

The following exercise goes through the treatment program one phase at a time.

Exercise 21

PHASE ONE

1. In primary standstill, you'll see no _____ complexes on the monitor.   QRS

2. But _____ waves may persist.   P

3. Remember, you'll treat the _____ and not the monitor.   patient

4. So go _____ the patient before doing anything else.   examine

5. This patient will _____ be conscious, will have _____ pulses, _____ blood pressure, and have _____ pupils.   not, no, no dilated

6. Can you differentiate between ventricular standstill and ventricular fibrillation at the bedside? _____   no

7. How can you differentiate between them? _____   with an ECG or monitor

PHASE TWO

1. Primary ventricular standstill will usually develop unexpectedly. (True/False)   False

2. What arrhythmias might precede it? _____ _____ or _____.   heart blocks bradyarrhythmias

3. Hopefully, these warning arrhythmias were recognized previously and your patient will have a prophylactic_____ _____ already in place if ventricular standstill develops.   transvenous pacemaker

4. If not, the first thing you should do is _____ _____. (It takes little time, requires no equipment, does no harm, and it may work.)   strike the chest with your fist

5. If this fails, _____ is essential to maintain circulation.   CPR

6. A doctor may insert a transthoracic needle through the chest directly into the _____ in an attempt to pace the heart.   heart

7. More likely, he may try to insert a _____ pacemaker.   transvenous

8. Pacing must be accomplished within _____ to _____ minutes. | 1, 2

9. The drug _____ may be helpful in restoring a heartbeat. | epinephrine or adrenalin

PHASE THREE

1. With ventricular standstill, _____ acidosis develops quickly because of the absence of oxygen. | lactic

2. IV _____ _____ should be given to correct this metabolic disorder. | sodium bicarbonate

PHASE FOUR

1. Patients who survive should be _____ as long as they have any heart block. | paced

2. Transvenous pacemakers should be left in place on a _____ basis to prevent recurrences. | standby

VENTRICULAR STANDSTILL PROCEDURE

Step 1. Recognition of problem. (Indications)

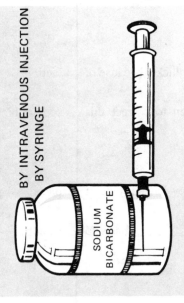

Step 2.

CODE 99

(or "DR. BLUE", etc.)

Step 3. Precordial thump.

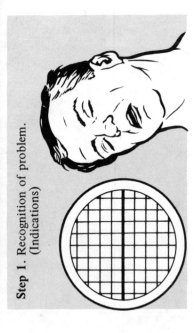

Step 4. External pacing.

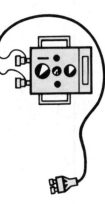

IF TRANSVENOUS PACEMAKER IS <u>NOT</u> IN PLACE, TRY EXTERNAL PACING:

1) <u>only</u> if immediately available

2) <u>only</u> for 1 minute if unsuccessful

Step 5. Cardiopulmonary resuscitation (CPR).

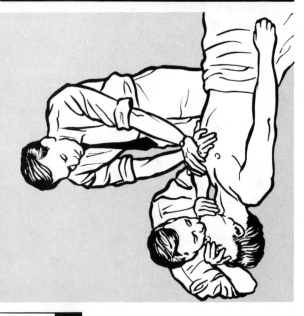

Step 6. Sodium bicarbonate.

BY INTRAVENOUS INJECTION BY SYRINGE

SODIUM BICARBONATE

Step 7. Prepare for transthoracic or transvenous pacing.

PULSE INDICATOR

RATE

MILLI-AMPS

Figure 13.12.

14

Electrical Treatment of Arrhythmias

TYPES OF CARDIAC PACING (*ICC, 4th ed., pp. 227-228*)

Sometimes the heart's electrical system is injured after an acute myocardial infarction and an artificial pacemaker is needed to keep the heart beating. In a sense, a pacemaker is a battery. It sends current to the heart by way of wires called catheter electrodes. Sounds simple, doesn't it?

Intensive Coronary Care, 4th ed., has only briefly touched upon external and transthoracic pacing as these methods are now seldom used. However, some hospital protocols may still require use of these pacemakers, so here is a quiz on them to try. (Don't be upset if you don't know all the answers.)

Exercise 1

1. Normally the ventricles contract in response to_____ stimuli   electrical
   originating within the heart.

2. External electrical stimulus can also be used to make the ventricles
   _____.   contract

3. This can be done with a _____.   pacemaker

4. Pacemaker impulses are generated by a _____.   battery

5. An outmoded way to conduct the battery's impulses to the heart is through an
   _____ placed on the chest wall.   electrode

6. This is called _____ pacing.   external

7. Another way is to pass a needle electrode through the chest wall directly into the
   _____.   myocardium

8. This is called _____ pacing.   transthoracic

9. Or electrodes can be passed into the right ventricle through _____.   veins

10. This is called _____ pacing.   transvenous

11. The three types of temporary pacing are _____, _____,
    and _____.   external, transthoracic transvenous

Exercise 2

1. External pacing (is/is not) usually successful. — is not

2. To be successful, it must be accomplished within _____ to _____ seconds. — 15, 30

3. Two disadvantages of external pacing are _____ and _____ _____. — pain, skin burns

4. If external pacing is attempted, the energy output dial should be set at its _____ level. — maximum

5. You should start _____ _____ within 1 minute. — cardiopulmonary resuscitation (CPR)

   Okay, we've given up on external pacing because it seldom works. What about transthoracic pacing?

6. The major advantage of transthoracic pacing is its _____ of application. — speed

7. To insert a transthoracic pacemaker, the doctor will need a _____ needle. — long #18 (an intracardiac needle)

8. The chest should be prepped around the _____ or _____ _____ _____. — 5th, 6th interspace near the middle of the chest

9. The doctor will insert the intracardiac needle into the ventricular wall, and a stainless steel _____ will then be threaded through the needle. — wire

10. The _____ is withdrawn and the _____ is left in the ventricular wall to serve as an electrode. — needle, wire

11. A second electrode is necessary. This ground electrode can be a _____ suture placed in the chest wall. — wire

12. The two wires are connected to the _____. — pacemaker

Now we consider transvenous pacing. It is used much more frequently and successfully than either external or transthoracic pacing. A transvenous pacing electrode can be inserted when the first warning signs of increasing heart block are seen. But the pacemaker doesn't have to be used for stimulating the heart unless it's needed, and the patients find the electrode no more (sometimes less) uncomfortable than an IV needle.

Exercise 3

1. In transvenous pacing the electrodes are passed through a _____ into the heart. — vein

2. The electrode passes through a peripheral vein into the _____ _____, to the right _____, and finally into the right _____. — vena cava atrium, ventricle

3. You connect the free end of the pacing catheter to a _____. — pacemaker

4. It's best to insert the transvenous pacing as a (preventive/emergency) measure. — preventive

5. Transvenous pacing is most often used to treat advancing forms of _____. — heart block

6. It can also be used to treat _____. — bradycardias

7. With extreme bradycardias, premature ventricular contractions are (more likely/less likely) to occur. — more likely

8. By (increasing/decreasing) the heart rate with a pacemaker, these PVCs may be eliminated. — increasing

9. This is called _____ the heart. — overdriving

PULSE GENERATORS (*ICC, 4th ed., pp. 228-230*)

We've got an electrode in place to allow stimulation of the heart. Now we have to send an electrical current to the electrode. The device that sends the current is called a

164

pacemaker or a pulse generator. It runs on batteries. This exercise reviews this magic little box.

Exercise 4

1. The simplest pacemaker uses a _____ rate pulse generator. | set or fixed

2. If you set the pacing rate at 60, the generator fires _____ times per minute. | 60

3. On the monitor you should see _____ pacemaker "blips" per minute. (See Figure 14.1, p. 228, (*ICC*, 4th ed.) | 60

4. After each pacing blip you should see a wide _____. | QRS

5. This QRS resembles a _____ pattern. | bundle branch block

6. If the heart beats by itself, the fixed-rate pacer (will/will not) fire anyway. | will

7. Thus, the pacemaker may _____ with the heart's natural impulses. | compete

8. As you remember, one of the dangers of PVCs is the _____-_____-_____ phenomenon, which can cause ventricular fibrillation. | R-on-T

9. Competition caused by pacing can also cause the _____-_____-_____ phenomenon if the pacing impulse strikes a T wave. | R-on-T

10. This, too, results in the potential threat of _____ _____. | ventricular fibrillation

"American ingenuity" came to the rescue, and the newer pacemakers use a *demand pulse generator.* How does this ingenious pacemaker operate?

Exercise 5

1. If a demand pacemaker senses a natural heartbeat, it (will/will not) fire. | will not

2. However, if the heart does not beat within a preset interval, the pacemaker will _____. | fire

3. When there is a natural, conducted heartbeat (R wave), the catheter tip transmits this information to a _____ device in the pacemaker. | sensing

4. When there is no natural heartbeat (no R wave), the pacemaker discharges an _____ _____ back to the heart. | electrical impulse

5. This type of pacemaker is called an R wave (inhibited/activated) pacemaker. | inhibited

6. The demand catheter has (1/2) function(s). | 2

7. It serves as an ECG electrode to (send/sense) natural beats and as a pacing catheter to (send/sense) electrical stimuli. | sense / send

8. The demand pacemaker is designed to avoid _____ _____, | competition with the natural heartbeat

9. And therefore prevent _____ _____. | ventricular fibrillation

PACING ELECTRODES (*ICC*, 4th ed., p. 230)

Now that we've talked about different kinds of pacemakers, let's discuss different kinds of electrodes.

Exercise 6

1. To complete an electrical circuit, the pacemaker needs (1/2) electrode(s). | 2

2. A unipolar catheter has (1/2) electrode(s) inside the heart, | 1

3. And one _____ the heart. | outside

4. The heart electrode is the (negative/positive) pole. | negative

165

5. The positive electrode is a wire suture in the _____. | skin

6. A bipolar catheter places (1/2) electrode(s) inside the heart. | 2

7. Both electrodes are encased inside the _____. | catheter

8. (Bipolar/unipolar) pacing is most successful. | bipolar

PACING TECHNIQUES (*ICC, 4th ed., pp. 230-235*)

We're ready now to learn about inserting and using a pacemaker. We'll stress the nursing role all the way through.

Exercise 7

1. The 3 veins generally used to insert a transvenous pacing electrode are
_____, _____, or _____. | antecubital, jugular, subclavian

2. Which vein is the least desirable? _____ | antecubital

3. The catheter is threaded from the vein into the _____ _____, to the right _____, to the right _____. | vena cava atrium, ventricle

4. Before the catheter is inserted, you'll need supplies for _____ and _____ the skin. | cleaning draping

5. Catheter insertion is usually performed through a large, special _____. | needle

6. Or a _____-_____ incision may be needed. | cut-down

7. Thus, you should have a _____-_____ tray handy. | cut-down

8. The electrode catheter is passed from the _____, _____, or _____ vein into the _____ _____, into the _____, through the _____ valve, and into the _____. | antecubital, jugular subclavian, superior vena cava, right atrium, tricuspid right ventricle

9. The doctor may use _____ to see where the catheter is going. | fluoroscopy

10. In the CCU, the doctor can follow the catheter by means of an _____. | ECG

11. Then you (would/would not) attach 4 limb leads to the patient. | would

12. The free end of the catheter attaches to the _____ lead of the ECG with an alligator clip. | chest (or V)

13. The tracing is called an _____ ECG. | intracavitary

14. The pacemaker has _____ terminals for connecting the catheter. | 2

15. These are marked _____ and _____. | negative, positive

16. With a unipolar catheter, insert the free end into the (negative/positive) terminal. | negative

17. The positive terminal would be connected to a _____ _____ _____. | wire skin suture

18. With a bipolar catheter, either wire can be connected to negative or positive terminals. (True/False) | True

When the catheter is in and attached to the pacemaker, how fast should the heart be paced?

19. The pacing rate must be (faster/slower) than the existing heart rate. | faster

20. If the pacing rate is too fast, the patient may complain of _____. | angina

21. Too fast rates may also (decrease/increase) ventricular filling and thus (decrease/increase) cardiac output. | decrease, decrease

22. Too slow rates might permit _____ arrhythmias to develop. | ectopic

In addition to the rate dial, your pacemaker will have an energy or intensity setting. How is this set?

23. The (lowest/highest) electrical setting that causes a contraction is the threshold level. | lowest

24. Settings lower than threshold (will/will not) cause contractions. | will not

25. Settings higher than threshold (will/will not) cause stronger contractions. | will not

26. To find the threshold level, start with the (lowest/highest) setting on the dial. | lowest

27. Increase the setting until you see a _____ with each pacing impulse. | QRS

28. This is the _____ level. | threshold

29. The usual level is less than _____ milliamperes. | 2

30. The threshold level (does/does not) vary with time and electrode contact. | does

31. Thus the energy setting is usually set (higher/lower) than threshold. | higher

32. This energy setting is scaled in _____. | milliamperes

33. The pacemaker is usually left in the heart as long as _____ _____ persist. | heart block or other arrhythmias

34. This is seldom over _____ days. | 10

35. But it may be left in a _____ longer, "just in case." | week

You can bet that your patient or his family will ask you, "Nurse, how long will this pacemaker be left in?" While the patient's doctor will decide, you should have some idea of what to expect.

PACING PROBLEMS (*ICC, 4th ed., pp. 235-236*)

Pacemakers can save lives, but they can also cause some problems. As with any machine, all sorts of things can go wrong, and you need to know about these problems.

Exercise 8

1. To pace effectively, the electrode tip should touch the inner _____ of the ventricle. | wall (endocardium)

2. If it doesn't, pacing _____ may occur. | failure

3. This type of pacing failure is called _____ of _____. | loss, capture

4. Loss of capture means that the pacemaker is firing but the heart isn't _____ in response to it. | beating

5. In this situation, the doctor may have to _____ the catheter. | reposition

6. In the meantime, you can try _____ _____. | changing the patient's position

7. For example, if the patient turned over in bed and capture is lost, try turning him _____. | back

8. Catheters inserted in the (arm/neck) are more prone to loss of capture. | arm

9. If the heart initiates its own beats between pacemaker-induced beats, we say _____ exists. | competition

10. Competition is more common with (fixed/demand) pacing. | fixed

11. However, a demand pacemaker may fire unnecessarily if the patient's QRS is too _____ to be sensed. | small

12. If you suddenly see no pacing blips on the monitor, the pacemaker (is/is not) functioning. | is not

13. Quickly, check the pacemaker to see if the pulse _____ (usually a flashing light) is working. | indicator

14. If the battery isn't firing, don't waste time. The problem then is with the battery, not the patient or electrode position. If this is the case, replace the _____. — battery

15. Make sure all connections are _____. — tight

16. Be ready to start _____ _____. — cardiopulmonary resuscitation

17. If your patient's chest muscles begin to twitch during pacing, the electrodes may have _____ the ventricle wall. — perforated

18. This may also cause contractions of the _____. — diaphragm

19. Perforation usually (does/does not) cause dangerous bleeding from the ventricle. — does not

20. If perforation occurs, the doctor will have to _____ the catheter. — reposition

21. Infection of the catheter insertion site can be minimized by _____ _____ during insertion and the use of _____ _____ afterwards. — aseptic technique, antibiotic ointment

22. After pacemaker insertion, watch the veins (especially in the arm) for signs of _____. — thrombophlebitis or inflammation

NURSING ROLE IN PACING (*ICC, 4th ed., pp. 236-238*)

Exercise 9

Dr. Hart says, "We're going to put in a pacemaker." What do you bring to the scene? Answer the following questions and then read the discussion that accompanies the answers. It will make this exercise more helpful if you can imagine yourself "flying" around collecting all these items while Dr. Hart impatiently taps his foot!

1. How do you prepare a conscious patient for an elective insertion?
   How about during an emergency?

2. What procedures do you follow to treat PVCs and ventricular fibrillation?

3. "Monitoring" the catheter during insertion requires:

4. Skin preparation requires:

5. Draping requires:

6. Catheter insertion requires:

7. Catheter securing requires:

8. While the doctor is busy inserting the catheter, who watches the ECG or monitor?

Answers and Discussion

1. Preparing the patient for an elective insertion means *explaining*. Emphasize the positive and relate it to the familiar. You might say something like: "You know, when you have an infection we can help your body by giving you a dose of penicillin or another antibiotic. Now, if your heart needs help, we can give it a 'dose' of pacemaker." You may frighten a patient who isn't comfortable with your terminology if you say: "This is a prophylactic measure which we will activate if you go into complete heart block to prevent your heart from going into ventricular fibrillation. It emits bursts of electricity that are conducted to your heart by . . ." Pretty scary stuff, right?

   Most hospitals require a "*permit*" for elective procedures such as this. Know your hospital's policy.

   In an emergency? *Try to save the patient's life first.* Someone should explain the procedure to the family, and some hospitals may obtain consent from family members to insert the pacemaker. If you're setting up for an emergency insertion, delegate the explanations and permission business to others.

2. PVCs and ventricular fibrillation during pacemaker insertion? Yes, they're both possible any time. Have a *patent IV* and *lidocaine* handy. Bring the *defibrillator* to the scene, plug it in, and screen it (if the patient is conscious) before the insertion is attempted.

3. For "monitoring" during an insertion you need an *ECG, limb leads,* and an *alligator clamp.* The ECG should be battery-operated; if not, be sure you ground it! Put the limb leads on the patient. After the catheter is inserted into the vein, connect the ECG chest lead to the catheter with an alligator clamp.

4. You'll need *skin cleaning and antiseptic supplies.* You'll have to find out what the doctor likes. Some want "that red stuff"; some like sprays; some swab it on. In an emergency, cleanse the skin with any antiseptic you have on hand, and don't worry.

5. *Drapes,* such as an "eye drape," small wound drape, or sterile towels, are needed. A sterile draw sheet, if you have one, turns the whole area into a "sterile" field.

6. *Cut-down set, local anesthetic, needle placement set*—don't forget the pacing catheters and the pacemaker! And just about now you'll be sending for size 8½ gloves instead of size 8. Once things get started, it's very handy if you can put on one sterile glove—then you can help in both the sterile field and with the unsterile pacemaker.

7. The catheter is in, you connect it, watch the monitor, and hooray! There's a QRS after every pacemaker blip. Now you'll need to secure the catheter: *sutures, tape, antibiotic ointment, and dressings.*

8. You do!

Exercise 10

The pacemaker is in; the doctor goes home. Who must make sure "all systems are go"? You, right? Now, suppose that your patient's monitor suddenly looks like this:

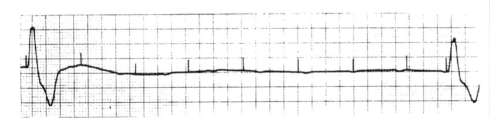

Figure 14.1.

What do you do?

1. Check the patient's _____ and _____ _____. pulse, blood pressure

2. _____ his position. Change

3. _____ the doctor. Notify

4. If necessary, start _____. CPR

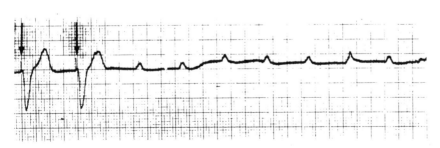

Figure 14.2.

169

Exercise 11

Another patient's monitor shows this tracing (Fig. 14.2). What do you do?

1. First, make sure catheter terminals are not _____ or _____.   disconnected, loose

2. Check the _____ _____ on the pacemaker to see if the battery is firing.   pulse indicator

3. If not, _____ the battery. (You should have a standby battery.)   replace

4. Start _____ if necessary.   CPR

5. _____ the doctor.   Notify

6. If you notice competition, you _____ the doctor.   notify

7. If you notice twitching of the chest muscles, you _____ the doctor.   notify

8. Twice a day, at least, check the insertion site for _____ or _____.   infection inflammation

MONITOR PRACTICE (*ICC, 4th ed., Chapter 14*)

See if you can interpret what the monitor tells you about pacemaker function. I've selected a series of monitor strips for us to analyze.

Exercise 12

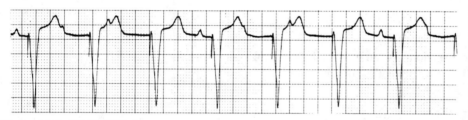

Figure 14.3. PATIENT 1.

This is a fixed-rate pacemaker.

1. Is it capturing?   yes

2. Is there any competition?   no

3. Is the pacemaker functioning well?   yes

4. What is the pacing rate?   about 70 beats/min

5. Are there any P waves?   yes

6. Do they have any relationship to the QRS complexes?   no

7. What type of heart block do you think the pacemaker is being used for?   third degree

Exercise 13

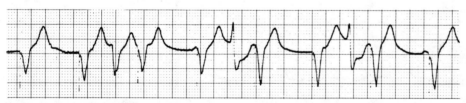

Figure 14.4. PATIENT 2.

1. Is it a fixed-rate or a demand pacemaker?   fixed-rate

2. Are there any natural heartbeats seen?   yes

3. Does the pacemaker recognize them?

no

4. What is the danger of this?

The pacing impulse may strike a T wave

5. This could result in _____ _____ .

ventricular fibrillation

6. What should you do?

Tell the doctor.

Exercise 14

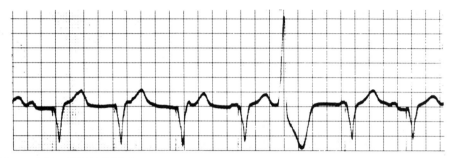

Figure 14.5. PATIENT 3.

1. What kind of pacemaker is this?

demand

2. Is it functioning well?

yes

3. What did the pacemaker do when it recognized a PVC?

It didn't fire, and reset itself.

Exercise 15

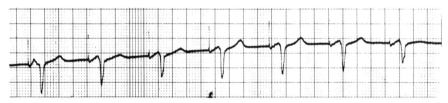

Figure 14.6. PATIENT 4.

1. Are the pacing spikes regular?

yes

2. Do the QRS complexes show the customary bundle branch pattern?

no

3. Why not?

The pacemaker is in the atrium; this is atrial pacing.

Exercise 16

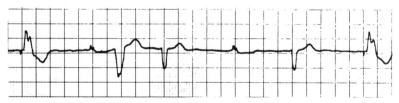

Figure 14.7. PATIENT 5.

1. The first and last beats on this strip show that pacemaker stimulus _____ the ventricles.

captures

2. But in between these two beats, the pacing stimulus produces no _____ .

response

3. There has been loss of _____ during this period.

capture

4. Is this dangerous? _____

yes

5. What should you do? _____

notify the doctor

171

6. What is the most likely cause of this problem? _____ _____.

      displacement of the catheter tip

7. What will have to be done? _____ _____.

      probably reposition the catheter

PRECORDIAL SHOCK (*ICC, 4th ed., p. 238*)

We'd better straighten out some terms before we study precordial shock. There are two uses of shock: 1) as an emergency life-saving measure; 2) as a therapeutic measure the doctor may elect to use rather than drug treatment in controlling arrhythmias. The first, *defibrillation*, refers to the emergency treatment of ventricular fibrillation, whereas the second, *cardioversion*, refers to a therapeutic measure used to correct some atrial and ventricular arrhythmias (but it is not used for ventricular fibrillation). Both types of shock are performed with the same machine, the defibrillator.

Exercise 17

1. One form of electric shock is called defibrillation. (True/False)

      True

2. Defibrillation is used to terminate _____ _____.

      ventricular fibrillation

3. Defibrillation is an emergency lifesaving measure. (True/False)

      True

4. Defibrillation uses a _____ voltage shock.

      high

5. It stops (all/some) of the heart's electrical activity for a fraction of a second.

      all

6. Then, hopefully, normal sinus rhythm reestablishes itself. (True/False)

      True

7. The chances for successful defibrillation (increase/decrease) with any delay in performing the procedure.

      decrease

8. Defibrillation is a term also used for elective treatment of arrhythmias. (True/False)

      False

9. The second form of precordial shock is called _____.

      cardioversion

10. Cardioversion can be used to terminate _____ as well as ventricular arrhythmias.

      atrial

11. Cardioversion is an elective, therapeutic measure. (True/False)

      True

12. The basic electrical principles of cardioversion and defibrillation (are/are not) the same.

      are

13. However, _____ must be used at a particular time in the cardiac cycle.

      cardioversion

14. _____ is not synchronized with any part of the cardiac cycle.

      Defibrillation

15. Both types of shock can be delivered by the same machine. (True/False)

      True

THE DEFIBRILLATOR (*ICC, 4th ed., p. 238*)

Now let's get acquainted with the defibrillator (when it's unplugged, please!)

Exercise 18

1. You're most likely to find (AC/DC) defibrillators in your hospital.

      DC

2. DC defibrillators can be used for (both/one) kind(s) of shock.

      both

3. When you turn the defibrillator on, it first (stores/delivers) electrical energy.

      stores

4. When you press the discharge switch, it (stores/delivers) electrical energy.

      delivers

5. There are three places you might find the discharge switch: on the machine, on the paddles, a foot switch. The most dangerous location is _____. (Someone may accidentally step on it.)

      foot switch

6. Where is the discharge switch on your defibrillator? — ???

7. The energy delivered by a defibrillator is measured in terms of _____ _____. — watt-seconds

8. The scale usually ranges from _____ to _____ watt-seconds. (This may vary slightly with different machines.) — 1, 400

9. What is the range on your defibrillator? — ???

10. The electrodes placed on the chest wall are usually called _____. — paddles

11. There is less likelihood of burning the patient's skin with (large/small) paddles. — large

12. Insulated handles on the paddles protect _____ from getting shocked. — you

13. Before defibrillating, apply a layer of _____ _____ to the defibrillator paddles. — conductive paste

SYNCHRONIZED AND NONSYNCHRONIZED SHOCK (*ICC, 4th ed., pp. 238-239*)

Before we begin the next section, do you remember the R-on-T phenomenon? If not, go back to *ICC*, 4th ed., review the ECG strip for the R-on-T pattern, and read the comments.

Exercise 19

1. An R-on-T type PVC can theoretically cause _____ _____. — ventricular fibrillation

2. Precordial shock striking on the T wave (could/could not) possibly cause ventricular fibrillation. — could

3. In treating atrial arrhythmias with shock, you (could/could not) possibly hit the T. — could

4. So you could possibly convert atrial arrhythmias to ventricular _____. — fibrillation

5. Would you ever want to do this? — NO, NO, NO

6. The T wave is in the (vulnerable/nonvulnerable) period in the cardiac cycle. — vulnerable

7. The nonvulnerable period is also called the _____ period. — refractory

8. The QRS is in the (vulnerable/refractory) period. — refractory

9. Synchronized shock is delivered in the (vulnerable/refractory) period. — refractory

10. The defibrillator does this by recognizing the _____ complex and firing at that time. — QRS

11. The synchronizer switch must be (on/off) for a defibrillator to sense the QRS wave. — on

12. In ventricular fibrillation, _____ complexes do not exist. — QRS

13. Thus, if the synchronizer is on, the machine (can/cannot) find an R wave to discharge on. — cannot

14. If you have the synchronizer on, can you treat ventricular fibrillation? — no

15. If you have the synchronizer on, can you treat atrial fibrillation? — yes

16. If you have the synchronizer *off*, can you treat ventricular fibrillation? — yes

17. If you have the synchronizer *off*, can you safely treat atrial fibrillation? — no

18. Do you fully understand questions 14-17?
(If not, reread this section in *ICC*, 4th ed., until you do.)

19. Ventricular fibrillation should be treated at the _____ energy setting. | highest or maximum

20. This is a maximum delivered energy of about _____ to _____ w/s. | 300, 350

21. In synchronized shock, the doctor determines the _____ _____ to use for a particular arrhythmia. | energy setting

SYNCHRONIZED SHOCK: CARDIOVERSION
(ICC, 4th ed., pp. 239-241)

Dr. Hart calls and says, "I'll be in within 15 minutes to use synchronized shock on the patient with atrial fibrillation." What do you do?

Exercise 20

1. First, _____ the procedure to the patient. | explain

2. Have the patient sign a _____. | permit or release

3. Bring the _____ to the bedside. | machine

(If your defibrillator has a built-in synchronizer, that's only one piece of equipment you'll need. If not, you'll need a defibrillator and a synchronizer, plus the cords to connect them.)

4. Emergency supplies you may need should be on your _____ _____. Bring it to the bedside. | crash cart

5. Supplies should include a syringe containing 100-mg _____. | lidocaine

6. Resuscitation equipment should include: _____, _____ _____, _____ _____. | airways, breathing bag, cardiac board

7. You should have an _____ line in place in this patient. | IV

8. Some type of _____ or sedation will be needed for the shock. | anesthetic

9. _____ the patient that sedation will make the procedure quite tolerable. | Reassure

If you bring this equipment, one piece at a time, and prepare and assemble it in the patient's room, you're going to scare him so badly that you may never need the synchronizer! Reduce the fuss and apprehension to a minimum.

Exercise 21

If your synchronizer is separate from your defibrillator, be sure not only to read the instructions for this machine, but to practice assembling the pieces. The doctors will expect you to set up the equipment; in fact, they may not be familiar with your hospital's synchronizer at all. These general concepts should apply to almost any kind of synchronizer:

1. You first turn the synchronizer switch _____. | on

2. The synchronizer needs an _____ wave to synchronize itself on. | R or QRS

3. If the patient's QRS is too _____, the synchronizer may not recognize it. | small or low

4. Adjust the gain dial to get sufficient _____ of the QRS. | height or voltage

5. Some synchronizers can be set to recognize (negative/positive/both) R waves. How about yours? | both

6. The doctor determines the _____ setting. | watt-second

7. Some type of short-acting _____ is usually used for elective shock. Be sure to find out what drugs you'll need for this. | anesthetic

8. Apply just the right amount of _____ _____ or _____ _____ to help prevent burns.

conductive jelly
electrode paste

9. Paste squishing out from beneath the paddles (can/cannot) cause sparks.

can

10. The paddles are placed so that the current will _____ the heart.

cross or traverse

11. The paddles must be pressed _____ against the skin.

firmly

12. The paddles must be held _____ and not tilted.

flat

13. Everyone must _____ _____ when the shock is delivered.

stand back

14. When the discharge switch is pressed, the synchronizer will fire on the _____ wave.

R

15. You will see the patient's muscles _____.

contract

16. The _____ will show if normal rhythm results.

monitor

17. You should have lidocaine ready in case _____ occur.

PVCs

18. Though it's unlikely, ventricular fibrillation may result. If it does, turn the synchronizer _____ and shock again.

off

DEFIBRILLATION (*ICC, 4th ed., pp. 241-242*)

Now that you've mastered synchronized shock, defibrillation is simple. Please realize that paddle placement and the precautions we've just discussed are the same for defibrillation or cardioversion.

Exercise 22

1. Ventricular fibrillation must be treated with _____.

defibrillation

2. Defibrillation should be done within _____ to _____ minutes after the onset of fibrillation.

1, 2

3. This means you _____ to the bedside if ventricular fibrillation occurs.

run, not walk

4. You (do/do not) have to wait for a doctor's order to defibrillate. (Unless your hospital policy says you must, which would be a shame.)

do not

5. You use the (maximum/minimum) energy setting.

maximum

6. This is usually _____ w/s, or _____ to _____ delivered w/s.

400, 300, 350

7. _____ _____ is applied between the paddles and skin.

Conductive jelly

8. If at first you don't succeed, _____ again!

shock

Exercise 23

Place an S in front of the terms that pertain to synchronized shock. Place a D in front of those that apply to defibrillation.

_____ elective

S

_____ maximum energy

D

_____ nonsynchronized

D

_____ cardioversion

S

_____ anesthesia

S

_____ two minutes

D

_____ ventricular fibrillation

D

175

_____ permit required   S

_____ minimum energy   S

_____ emergency   D

Exercise 24

To review all we have discussed about cardioversion and defibrillation, study the diagram on cardioversion on the next page and the diagram on defibrillation, Figure 14.9, p. 178. I'm sure you'll be able to perform these procedures when necessary.

CARDIOVERSION PROCEDURE

Step 1. Recognition of problem.

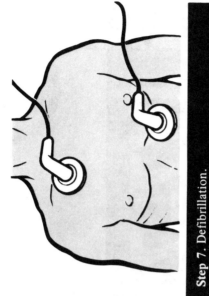

ECG

ATRIAL FLUTTER
ATRIAL FIBRILLATION
ATRIAL TACHYCARDIA
NODAL TACHYCARDIA
VENTRICULAR
TACHYCARDIA

Step 2. Prepare patient.

PSYCHOLOGICALLY
PHYSICALLY
LEGALLY

Step 3.

DEFIBRILLATOR <u>ON</u>
ON
OFF

SYNCHRONIZER <u>ON</u>
ON
OFF

Step 4. Set machine.

ZERO

+50 — 400+
RANGE
400

WATT-SECONDS

Step 5. Paddle positions.

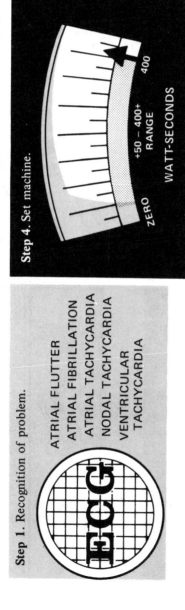

RIGHT STERNAL
BORDER
2nd SPACE

APEX

Step 6. Paddles in place, stand back!!!

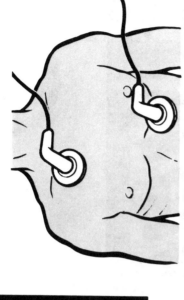

Step 7. Defibrillation.

Z-Z-ZAP!

Step 8. Success!

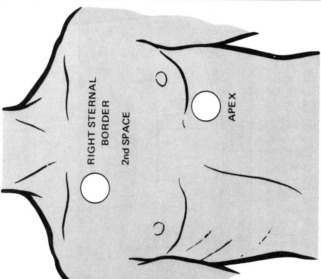

Figure 14.8.

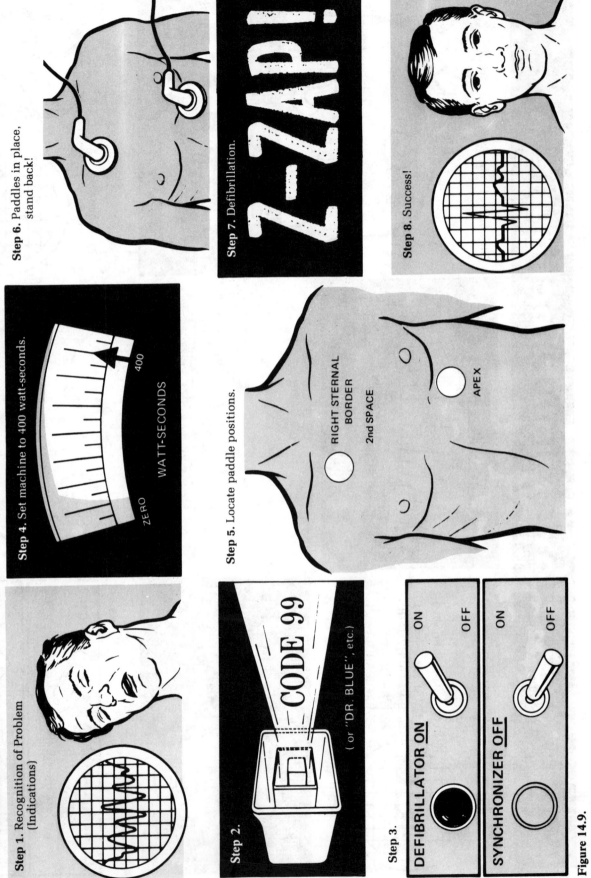

DEFIBRILLATION PROCEDURE

Step 1. Recognition of Problem (Indications)

Step 2.

CODE 99

(or "DR. BLUE", etc.)

Step 3.

DEFIBRILLATOR ON — ON OFF

SYNCHRONIZER OFF — ON OFF

Step 4. Set machine to 400 watt-seconds.

400

ZERO   WATT-SECONDS

Step 5. Locate paddle positions.

RIGHT STERNAL BORDER
2nd SPACE

APEX

Step 6. Paddles in place, stand back!

Step 7. Defibrillation.

Z-ZAP!

Step 8. Success!

Figure 14.9.

178

15

ECG Diagnosis of MI, Injury and Ischemia

Now if you're ready for some fun, let's begin our study of the 12-lead ECG. No matter how long you work in CCU, this is a skill you can continue to refine and expand. The more 12-lead ECGs (and their interpretations) that you study the more you will begin to recognize and identify. It's fun! *ICC*, 4th ed., has some marvelous illustrations; study and use them often. Ready? Let's go.

12-LEAD ECG (*ICC, 4th ed., pp. 243-244*)

Exercise 1

1. 12-lead ECGs are used to _____ the occurrence of an MI, _____ the site of the MI, and show the _____ of healing or the age of an MI.

   identify, localize
   stages

2. The 12-leads include: 3 standard _____ leads; 3 _____ leads; and 6 _____ leads.

   limb, augmented
   chest or precordial

3. A different classification lists 3 (bipolar/unipolar) and 9 (bipolar/unipolar).

   bipolar, unipolar

4. A bipolar lead measures the (actual/difference in) electrical potential between 2 electrodes.

   difference in

5. A (bipolar/unipolar) lead shows the actual electrical potential at the electrode sites.

   unipolar

6. The bipolar leads are _____.

   Leads I, II, III

7. The other 9 leads are _____.

   unipolar

BIPOLAR AND UNIPOLAR LEADS

Exercise 2

1. Do Leads I, II, and III make sense to you? If not, go back to Chapter 8, pg. 97 (4th ed.) Figure 8.2 of this workbook. As it suggests: take 6 pieces of tape, write one of the following on one of the pieces—I+, I−, II+, II−, III+, III−.

2. Place the tapes on your arms and legs (as ECG technicians place the electrodes) or on your shoulders and thigh for convenience. Place I− on your right shoulder and I+ on your left shoulder. Lead I records the difference in potential of depolarization coming from the right toward the left electrode.

3. Now place II− on your right shoulder and II+ on your left thigh. Again the difference in potential shows electrical forces traveling from negative (right arm) to positive (left thigh).

4. Finally place III− on your left shoulder and III+ on your left thigh. Lead III will show the electrical forces flowing from left shoulder to left thigh as a positive deflection.

5. Answer again the questions in Exercise 3, pg. 97.

6. Now can you "see" what the three positive limb electrodes are seeing? Look at some of the R waves in actual ECGs. The higher the R wave, the greater the difference in electrical potential sensed by the positive electrode. All negative waves were "traveling away from" the positive electrode.

Exercise 3

On to the unipolar leads and measurement of *actual* (rather than the difference in) electrical potentials at electrode sites.

1. Now you need to imagine the _____ being the center of Einthoven's triangle.

    heart

2. Next we assume that the electrical forces of the standard limb leads are equal to _____. (Canceling each other out is the way I think of it.)

    zero

3. So if the center of our triangle has no electrical force (zero), the exploring (recording) electrode will show the (actual/difference in) electrical potential at its site.

    actual

4. These unipolar electrodes (do/do not) use the same 3 limbs.

    do

5. The unipolar voltages are very low and must be electrically _____.

    augmented

6. Thus these leads are called the _____ unipolar leads.

    augmented

7. They are designated: aVR, (augmented _____ _____ arm); aVL, (_____ unipolar _____ arm); aVF, (augmented unipolar _____ _____).

    unipolar right
    augmented, left
    left leg ("foot" makes better sense!)

8. That wasn't so bad, was it? Now we have only 6 more unipolar leads; these are recorded from the _____.

    chest or precordium

9. The ECG technician (or you) moves an electrode across the _____ to record the (actual/difference in) electrical potential coming toward the electrode.

    chest
    actual

10. There are (3/6/9/12) chest leads.

    six

11. These leads are called (c/v) leads, and they move from (left to right/right to left).

    v, right to left

Exercise 4

1. Fill in the blanks in the diagram below:

Bipolar Leads	Unipolar Extremity Leads	Unipolar Chest Leads
_____	_____	_____
_____	_____	_____
_____	_____	_____
		_____
		_____
		_____

I	aVR	V1
II	aVL	V2
III	aVF	V3
		V4
		V5
		V6

180

DIAGNOSIS OF ACUTE MI (*ICC, 4th ed., pp. 244-248*)

Exercise 5

1. The three zones of an acute MI are:
   Zone 1: _____, Zone 2: _____, Zone 3: _____.
   (Memorize these.) — necrosis, injury, ischemia

2. The most severely damaged is zone _____, which is the zone of _____. — 1, necrosis

3. This shows on an ECG by changes in the (Q/ST/T) wave. — Q

4. What are the changes? — deep, wide Q

5. Can you explain this? — ?

6. Let's try. The electrode is looking through a "window" of (dead/active) muscle. So it records electrical activity going (away from it/toward it). This activity is actually the first part of the _____ depolarizing. (Remember, a force going away from an electrode records as (negative/positive) on the ECG. — dead / away / septum / negative

7. The Q waves of an acute MI occur after an MI (within an hour/ within days/both/neither). — both

8. Zone 2 of an acute MI is the area of _____. — injury

9. Zone 2 shows on an ECG by changes in the (Q/ST/T). — ST

10. The ST segment may be (elevated/depressed/both/neither). — both

11. If the ECG lead faces the injured area, the ST will be _____. — elevated

12. Depressed STs are also called _____ changes. — reciprocal

13. Elevated STs are convex and sometimes called a _____ ST. — coved

14. Coved STs show in leads (facing/away from) the injury. — facing

15. Zone 3 of an MI is the area of _____. — ischemia

16. Zone 3 shows on an ECG by changes in the (Q/ST/T). — T

17. The T waves may be _____ and sharply _____. — inverted, pointed

18. T wave changes (may/may not) be caused by things other than an MI. — may

LOCALIZING THE MI (*ICC, 4th ed., pp. 248-256*)

Exercise 6

1. With an acute transmural MI, all 3 zones (may/may not) be seen on the ECG. — may

2. So on an ECG you might find changes in _____, _____, and _____ waves. — Q, ST, T

3. Do all 3 changes need to be present for the diagnosis of an MI? — no

4. The ECG can tell you if the MI is an anterior, posterior, or inferior MI. (True/False) — true

5. Why does it matter to you where the MI is located? — prognosis and complications correlate with the site

6. Once again, the acute MI ECG pattern consists of: _____, _____, and _____.
   (Memorize this, you'll use it in Exercise 7 and in "diagnosing" MIs.) — deep Q waves elevated ST segments, inverted T waves

WHERE'S THE MI?

Exercise 7

One of the favorite games in CCU is called "Where's His MI?" It's a thrill to "diagnose" a 12-lead ECG and find out the cardiologist's diagnosis agrees with yours!

It takes lots of practice. To begin with, read pp. 249 and 255 in *ICC*, 4th ed., very carefully. Exercise 7 puts the material into a handy chart. Choose your answers from those given below. I suggest you photocopy the blank chart for extra practice. When you know the answer on the chart, then practice using the chart with real 12-lead ECGs and look for the changes in the leads specified.

Choices for answers in Exercise 7:

Characteristics and Complications Choices:

Higher incidence of heart block

Higher death rate

Higher incidence of pump failure

More frequently involves AV node

Involves larger pump mass

Electrocardiographic changes:

(Choices include all ECG leads)

Leads I, II, III

aVL, aVF, aVR

V1-V6

ANTERIOR MI	INFERIOR MI
Characteristics and Complications	
1. _____	1. _____
2. _____	2. _____
3. _____	
Electrocardiographic Changes	
Acute MI pattern	*Acute MI pattern*
1. Extensive Anterior MI:	1. Inferior MI:
_____	_____
_____	_____
_____	_____
2. Anteroseptal MI:	2. Inferolateral MI:
_____	* _____
_____	_____
_____	_____
3. Anterolateral MI:	* _____
_____	* _____
_____	*= ST, T changes

Answers

ANTERIOR MI	INFERIOR MI
Characteristics and Complications	
1. Higher death rate	1. Higher incidence of heart block
2. Involves larger muscle mass	2. More frequently involves AV node
3. Higher incidence of pump failure	
Electrocardiographic Changes	
Acute MI pattern	*Acute MI pattern*
1. Extensive Anterior MI:	1. Inferior MI:
Lead I	Lead II
aVL	Lead III
all V leads	aVF
2. Anteroseptal MI:	2. Inferolateral MI:
Lead I	*Lead I
aVL	Lead II
V1–V4	Lead III
3. Anterolateral MI:	aVF
Lead I	*aVL
aVL	*V5–V6
V4—V6	* = ST, T changes

STAGES OF AN MI (*ICC, 4th ed., p. 257*)

Exercise 8

1. In Exercise 7 we learned the acute MI patterns in specific ECG leads that help us identify the _____ of an MI.

    location

2. The 12-lead ECG also shows the stages of _____ of an MI.

    healing

3. Three stages shown by the ECG are: _____, _____, and _____.

    acute, recent
    old

4. As you know, the acute MI pattern is _____, _____, _____.

    deep Q waves, elevated STs, inverted Ts

5. When_____ and_____ return to normal (or stabilize), the MI is in the recent stage.

    ST, T

6. The "old" MI retains the _____ changes.

    Q

7. Pathological Q waves are wider than _____ second and deeper than _____ mm.

    0.04, 4

NONTRANSMURAL MIs (*ICC, 4th ed., pp. 260-261*)

Exercise 9

1. A nontransmural MI (does/does not) extend clear through the myocardium.

   does not

2. Nontransmural MIs produce only small patchy areas of _____ in the muscle.

   necrosis

3. Thus, the necrosis pattern of zone I, the _____ wave changes, are not found in the ECGs.

   Q

4. Sometimes the only ECG change will be in the _____.

   T

5. So nontransmural MIs may be called _____ _____ infarctions.

   T wave

6. Anterior nontransmural ECG changes occur in leads _____, _____, and ____ __ _____.

   I, aVL
   all V leads

7. Inferior nontransmural ECG changes occur in leads _____, _____, and _____.

   II, III
   aVF

8. The above are the same as in transmural MIs (see Exercise 7). (True/False)

   True

9. T waves changes can occur for reasons other than an MI. (True/False)

   True

10. Old nontransmural MIs can be identified by ECG changes. (True/False)

    False

ECG CHANGES IN ANGINA PECTORIS
(*ICC, 4th ed., pp. 262-264*)

Exercise 10

1. The underlying cause of angina pectoris is a transient myocardial _____.

   ischemia

2. Ischemia of angina shows in _____ depression (*not* elevation), and sometimes in _____ wave changes.

   ST
   T

3. This (is/is not) the same as the zones of injury change in acute MIs. (Review Exercise 5 and study *ICC*, 4th ed., p. 248 to see why.)

   is not

4. Variant angina pectoris, also called _____ involves pain (at rest/during exertion).

   Prinzmetal's, at rest

5. The underlying cause of variant angina is _____ _____ _____. (Compare to Question 1)

   coronary artery spasm

6. This causes _____ segment (elevation/depression) on the ECG.

   ST, elevation

7. Can you differentiate between stable angina pectoris and variant angina on the ECG? (See Questions 2 & 6).

   yes

8. After a period of angina, the ECG changes should promptly return to normal (the baseline). (True/False)

   True

9. Failure to return to normal probably indicates _____ _____.

   an acute MI, not just angina

EXERCISE (STRESS) TESTING (*ICC, 4th ed., p. 265*)

Exercise 11

1. Stress testing may be done to confirm the diagnosis of _____.

   angina

2. Exercise is used to increase the myocardial _____ demand.

   oxygen

3. ECGs taken before, during and after exercise show myocardial _____ during exercise if the test is positive.

   ischemia

4. This is shown by _____ _____ on the ECG.

   ST depression

5. Stress testing (is/is not) entirely reliable.

   is not

16

Antiarrhythmic Drugs

MECHANISMS OF DRUG ACTION
(ICC, 4th ed., p. 267)

Antiarrhythmic drugs alter automaticity, excitability, and conductivity functions of cardiac cells. Are you confused? Perhaps it will help if you try writing your own definitions of these terms without checking the answers that follow. Just try for the general ideas, not necessarily word-for-word perfection.

Exercise 1

1. Define automaticity:

2. Define excitability:

3. Define conductivity:

Answers

1. *Automaticity* is the ability of certain cells within the heart to spontaneously *initiate* electrical impulses.

2. *Excitability* is the ability of cardiac cells to *respond* to stimulation.

3. *Conductivity* is the velocity at which impulses are transmitted through the specialized fibers of the conduction system.

Exercise 2

Shall we try a few more questions to be sure you've got the three mechanisms straight?

1. Drugs can affect the threshold level at which cardiac cells will respond to a stimulus. (True/False)

   True

2. The threshold level of stimulation relates to _____.

   excitability

3. Slow or accelerated transmission velocities relate to _____.

   conductivity

4. In other words, we're talking about how _____ an electrical wave travels.

   fast

5. Drugs can affect the velocity at which impulses travel through the conduction system. (True/False)

   True

6. The rate of spontaneous firing of cardiac cells relates to_____. | automaticity

7. Drugs can affect the rate at which pacemaker cells discharge their impulses. (True/False) | True

Exercise 3

Table 16.1 identifies the 3 mechanisms of antiarrhythmic action. You won't be able to fill in all the blanks at this stage, but as you continue to work in CCU you'll be able to complete the table as you learn more about antiarrhythmic drugs. Two blanks have been filled in to help you get started and a partially completed table follows with answers from *ICC*, 4th ed.

Table 16.1. Summary of Mechanisms of Antiarrhythmic Action

	Automaticity	*Excitability*	*Conductivity*
Definition:	Ability to initiate impulses spontaneously		
Increase caused by:			
Decrease caused by:			
Increase leads to:	Ectopics and tachycardias		
Decrease leads to:			
Drugs that increase:			
Drugs that decrease:			

Answers to Table 16.1. Summary of Mechanisms of Antiarrhythmic Action

	Automaticity	*Excitability*	*Conductivity*
Definition:	Ability to initiate impulses spontaneously	Ability to respond to stimulation (decrease in threshold level = increase in excitability)	Velocity at which impulses are transmitted
Increase caused by:		Low potassium	
Decrease caused by:		Inadequate myocardial perfusion	
Increase leads to:	Ectopics and tachycardias	Rapid rate arrhythmias repetitive firing	
Decrease leads to:	Sinus bradycardia	Normal impulse will not evoke a response	
Drugs that increase:	Atropine isoproterenol		Atropine isoproterenol
Drugs that decrease:	Lidocaine quinidine procainamide beta-blockers		Digitalis quinidine procainamide

186

CLASSIFICATION OF ANTIARRHYTHMIC DRUGS
(*ICC, 4th ed., pp. 267-269*)

ICC, 4th ed. categorizes antiarrhythmic drugs into 4 groups.

1. Drugs that act directly on cardiac cells.

2. Drugs that act indirectly on cardiac cells.

3. Drugs with a combined action.

4. Calcium blocking agents.

Exercise 4

Drugs can have a direct action on cardiac cells. Let's diagram the way in which anti-arrhythmic drugs work directly on the cardiac cell. Complete Figure 16.1; it begins with an electrical impulse: — — — — — ZAP! After the impulse strikes a cardiac cell there is an exchange of ions. Show the exchange of ions during depolarization and repolarization.

Figure 16.1.

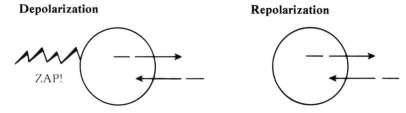

Depolarization
K ⟶
⟵——Na
Repolarization
Na ⟶
⟵——K

Exercise 5

Now take this little cardiac cell and hook it up to 2 tiny (micro) electrodes. This will produce a *transmembrane action potential* from that cell. We'll take the ZAP! from Figure 16.1 and assume it's strong enough to exceed the cell's threshold level (the point at which the cell will respond). Now let's see exactly what happens next.

Complete the labels on Figure 16.2, as you follow the instructions on the next page. (The action flows from left to right as you complete the diagram.)

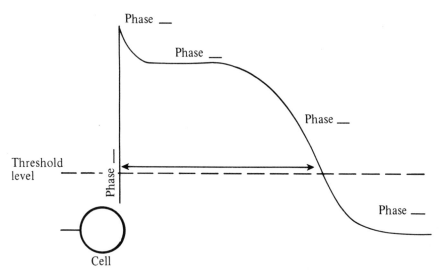

Figure 16.2.

187

1. ⋀⋀⋀ ZAP the cell gets hit. Draw the electrical impulse hitting the cell.

2. Show the K and Na exchange in the cell using arrows.

3. The sharp upstroke on our "ECG" is Phase _____, this is _____-polarization. (Fill in blanks here and on the diagram.)

4. The cell then goes through _____ -polarization; this includes Phases _____ through _____.

5. The potential returns to the baseline in Phase _____.

6. The cell cannot respond to another stimulus during the *Effective Refractory Period*. Show where it begins and ends on the diagram.

	0, de
	re, 1
	3
	3
	1-2

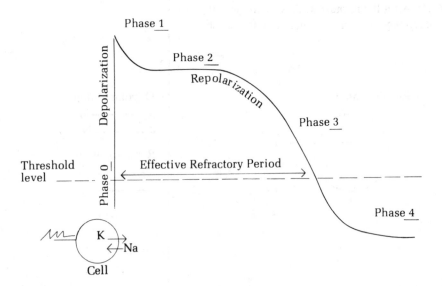

Answers to Figure 16.2.

Exercise 6

The next questions also relate to Figure 16.2.

1. Antiarrhythmic drugs that act directly on cardiac cells _____ the phases of the transmembrane action potential. — alter (change or affect)

2. These drugs work especially by changing the _____ _____ _____. (Find it on your diagram.) — effective refractory period (ERP)

3. During the ERP a cell (can/cannot) accept another stimulus. — cannot

4. Antiarrhythmic drugs can change the _____ of the ERP. — duration

Exercise 7

Some drugs act *indirectly* on the heart by stimulating or blocking the autonomic nervous system activity.

1. The autonomic nervous system includes the _____ and the _____ nervous systems. — sympathetic parasympathetic

2. To differentiate these: the_____ nervous system is sympathetic with you when you're in danger. (It gears you up to go-go-go!) — sympathetic

3. If you think of the sympathetic nervous system as the accelerator, then the _____ nervous system becomes the brakes. — parasympathetic

4. The increased parasympathetic action (slows down/speeds up) the heart. — slows down

188

5. Another name for the parasympathetic fibers that we're talking aout is _____. | vagus

6. Drugs can act on the autonomic nervous system in 4 ways.
   They can _____ the sympathetic nervous system. | stimulate
   They can _____ the sympathetic nervous system. | block
   They can _____ the parasympathetic nervous system. | stimulate
   They can _____ the parasympathetic nervous system. | block

7. Or, using different terminology for the last two:
   They can _____ vagal activity. | stimulate
   They can _____ vagal activity. | block

Exercise 8 (*ICC, 4th ed., pp. 268-269*)

Table 16.2 shows drug actions you can expect from various drugs. Fill in the blank columns using (↑) for increase, (↓) for decrease, and (⊖) for no effect.

Table 16.2. Classification of Drugs by Action

Drug	Heart rate	Conductivity	Force of Contraction	
			Atrial	Ventricular
Stimulates Sympathetic				
Stimulates Vagus				
Blocks Sympathetic				
Blocks Vagus				

Answers to Table 16.2. Classification of Drugs by Action

Drug	Heart rate	Conductivity	Force of Contraction	
			Atrial	Ventricular
Stimulates Sympathetic	↑	↑	↑	↑
Stimulates Vagus	↓	↓	↓	⊖
Blocks Sympathetic	↓	↓	↓	↓
Blocks Vagus	↑	↑	↑	⊖

Exercise 9: Combined Action

1. The drug _____ _____ is the best example of this group. | bretylium tosylate

2. It has (direct/indirect/both) actions on cardiac cells. | both

3. It (increases/decreases) the refractory period and (increases/decreases) excitability. | increases, decreases

189

Exercise 10: Calcium Blocking Agents

1. Calcium blocking agents are used primarily to treat _____ _____.   angina pectoris

2. They do this by relieving _____ _____ spasm.   coronary artery

3. They also block the entry of _____ into the cells.   calcium

4. Verapamil, a Ca blocker, slows conduction through the _____ _____ by increasing the refractory period.   AV node

5. Thus it is useful in controlling _____ tachycardias and slowing the ventricular rate in _____ _____.   supraventricular
atrial fibrillation

6. Two brands of verapamil you might find are _____ or _____.   Calan, Isoptin

INDIVIDUAL ANTIARRHYTHMIC DRUGS
(ICC, 4th ed., pp. 269-285)

QUINIDINE

Exercise 11: *USES*

1. Quinidine is most often used to treat _____ fibrillation and _____ ectopic beats.   atrial
ventricular

2. Quinidine is usually the first "drug of choice" for ventricular ectopics. (True/False)   False

Exercise 12: *ACTIONS*

Use the information in *ICC*, 4th ed., to complete as much as you can of Table 16.3, the Drug Action Chart. As we study *each* antiarrhythmic drug, you will be referred to Table 16.3. Complete as much of the chart as you can. Continue to fill in the chart as you work in CCU and as your knowledge of drugs grows. The chart appears on p. 205 in this chapter. The answers to the Drug Action Chart appear at the end of this chapter. Then try these questions without referring to *ICC*, 4th ed., or your chart.

1. Quinidine acts directly on the cell. (True/False)   True

2. Quinidine also (blocks/stimulates) the (vagus/sympathetic) nervous system.   blocks, vagus

3. Acting directly, it _____ automaticity.   decreases

4. It _____ excitability (especially atrial).   decreases

5. It _____ conduction, especially at the AV node.   slows

6. Unfortunately, it _____ the strength of myocardial contractility.   decreases

7. Thus, it _____ stroke volume and cardiac output.   decreases

8. The vagal blocking may cause the heart rate to _____,   increase

9. and conduction time to _____.   decrease

10. The vagal blocking effect may counteract the direct cellular effect. (True/False)   True

Exercise 13: *ADMINISTRATION AND DOSAGE*

Study the material in *ICC*, 4th ed., then see how much of Table 16.4, Drug Administration and Dosage Chart, you can complete. You will be using this chart for each drug's administration and dosage in much the same way as you use Table 16.3 to compile information on each drug's action. Use arrows for increase and decrease on both tables. The answers to Table 16.4 appear at the end of Chapter 16.

Exercise 14: *CONTRAINDICATIONS*

1. Two contraindications to quinidine you might note on the ECG are _____ _____ and _____ _____ _____.

   wide QRS, advanced AV block

2. Renal disease as shown by an elevated _____ might also be a contraindication to starting quinidine therapy.

   BUN

Exercise 15: *SIDE EFFECTS: CARDIAC*
(*Use Table 16.3 to answer*)

1. Quinidine's overall direct effect is one of _____ myocardial contractility.

   decreasing

2. Thus it may cause or exaggerate _____ _____.

   heart failure

3. Quinidine _____ conductivity through the AV node and can lead to AV _____.

   slows block

4. Toxic doses cause _____ _____ or _____ _____.

   ventricular tachycardia ventricular fibrillation

Exercise 16: *SIDE EFFECTS: SYSTEMIC*

The doctor has ordered 400 mg quinidine every 6 hours for your patient, Mr. Kardiak. What systemic reactions would you watch for? Which are most common?

1. Gastrointestinal system:

   nausea and vomiting, diarrhea

2. Vision/hearing:

   blurred vision, tinnitus, deafness

3. Allergies:

   fever, rashes

4. Which of the three are most common?

   gastrointestinal symptoms

5. You'd also watch your patient's monitor closely for two ECG changes (as well as rate changes); they are _____ _____ and _____ _____.

   widened QRS, AV block

6. Mr. Kardiak's serum quinidine level is 7 mg/liter; you know the desired level is _____ to _____ per liter. Do you call this to the doctor's attention? _____

   5, 7, Yes

7. Toxic levels are usually above _____ mg/liter.

   8

PROCAINAMIDE

Exercise 17: *USES*

1. If you can't find procainamide in the medicine cupboard, what other name would you look for? _____

   Pronestyl

2. Procainamide can be used for: (bradyarrhythmias/PVCs/tachyarrhythmias).

   PVCs, tachyarrhythmias

3. Procainamide may be used in treating PVCs when _____ fails.

   lidocaine

4. It may be used for supraventricular tachycardias when _____ cannot be used.

   quinidine

Exercise 18: *ACTIONS*

Use the information from *ICC*, 4th ed., to complete as much of Table 16.3 as you can. Then try these.

1. Procainamide _____ automaticity.

   decreases

2. It _____ excitability.

   decreases

3. It _____ conductivity.

   decreases

4. It _____ contractility.

   decreases

5. It is a myocardial (stimulant/depressant).

    depressant

6. Then why on earth do we use it?

    to control arrhythmias, especially PVCs

7. Is it usually the drug of choice in treating arrhythmias?

    No

Exercise 19: *ADMINISTRATION AND DOSAGE*

Study the material in *ICC*, 4th ed., and complete as much of Table 16.4 as you can.

Exercise 20: *CONTRAINDICATIONS*

The doctor is considering starting Mr. Kardiak on procainamide, and asks you to check his ECG.

1. You look especially for:

    AV block or intraventricular conduction defects

2. Before you give the first dose, what question might you ask Mr. Kardiak?

    Are you allergic to the novocaine your dentist uses? Or have you ever been allergic to the shots they use to numb the skin when they sew up a cut?

Exercise 21: *SIDE EFFECTS: CARDIAC*

1. Procainamide _____ conductivity.

    decreases

2. It can cause _____ or _____ heart block.

    AV, intraventricular

3. It _____ myocardial contractility.

    depresses

4. So it may cause or aggravate _____ _____.

    heart failure

5. Its vagal effect is to _____ heart rate.

    increase

6. This vagolytic action could possibly cause _____ _____.

    ventricular tachycardia

Exercise 22

Mr. Kardiak is now on a Pronestyl drip of about 125 mg/hour. (Poor man!) What do you watch for?

1. You measure the width of the _____ on his monitor strip.

    QRS

2. If the QRS increases more than _____%, you notify the doctor.

    50

3. Also, an increased _____ interval would make you call the doctor.

    PR

Exercise 23: *SIDE EFFECTS: SYSTEMIC*

1. The order for checking Mr. Kardiak's vital signs reads every 4 hours. You've just started his Pronestyl drip. Comment?

    Check his BP more often while the drug is being administered

2. Why? Because Pronestyl can cause serious _____.

    hypotension

3. Gastrointestinal reactions might include:

    anorexia, nausea, vomiting, abdominal pain, diarrhea, bitter taste in the mouth

4. Patients on long-term procainamide may develop a syndrome similar to _____ _____.

    lupus erythematosus

NORPACE

Exercise 24: *USES*

1. Norpace's generic name is _____.
   (That's why we'll call it Norpace.)

   Disopyramide

2. Norpace may be used to control the ventricular arrhythmias: _____ _____.

   PVCs and ventricular tach

3. It also helps terminate supraventricular arrhythmias: _____ _____ _____.

   sv. tachycardias atrial tach, atrial flutter, atrial fibrillation

Exercise 25: *ACTIONS*

Use the information from *ICC*, 4th ed., to complete as much of Table 16.3 as you can. Then try these:

1. Norpace's effects are similar to the effects of _____.

   quinidine

2. However, paradoxically, it can increase the ventricular response in _____ _____ or _____ _____.

   atrial flutter, atrial fibrillation

Exercise 26: *ADMINISTRATION AND DOSAGE*

Study the material in *ICC,* 4th ed., and complete as much of Table 16.4 as you can.

Exercise 27: *CONTRAINDICATIONS*

You admit an elderly man on the night shift. You know his doctor may use Norpace.

1. While examining the man, you're looking for signs or symptoms of _____ _____.

   heart failure, even MI

2. You'll question him about any _____ _____, _____ _____ or _____.

   urinary problems prostate trouble, glaucoma

Exercise 28: *SIDE EFFECTS*

1. Norpace's most serious side effect is _____ _____ _____.

   congestive heart failure

2. With high drug blood levels, it can cause _____ tachycardias.

   ventricular

3. Systemic effects you'd watch for include: _____ _____.

   dry mouth, blurry vision difficulty voiding, constipation

4. Then you might see: _____ _____.

   chills, fever, skin lesions, joint, muscle, and pleuritic pain

LIDOCAINE

Exercise 29: *USES*

1. Quick, get the lidocaine! The bottle or syringe you pick up might say _____; it's the same thing.

   xylocaine

2. Lidocaine is used to control _____ and _____ _____.

   PVCs, ventricular tachycardia

3. Lidocaine is not usually the drug of choice in treating ventricular ectopics. (True/False)

   False

Exercise 30: ACTIONS

Use the information in *ICC*, 4th ed., to complete as much of Table 16.3 as you can. Then try these.

1. Lidocaine _____ automaticity, especially in the _____-_____ _____.

   decreases, His Purkinje system

2. Lidocaine _____ the excitability threshold.

   raises

3. The excitability threshold is the point at which a cell will _____.

   depolarize

4. Thus, with lidocaine the ventricles are (more/less) likely to initiate or propagate ectopic beats.

   less

5. Lidocaine is commonly used to treat atrial tachyarrhythmias. (True/False)

   False

6. Why not? Because lidocaine has _____ or _____ effect on the atria.

   little, no

7. Lidocaine (does/does not) affect conduction velocity.

   does not

8. Lidocaine (does/does not) cause AV and intraventricular disturbances.

   does not (except very large doses)

9. Lidocaine has (little/great) effect on myocardial contractility.

   little

10. It has (little/great) effect on peripheral vascular resistance.

    little

11. It (does/does not) usually affect cardiac output and blood pressure.

    does not

12. Lidocaine begins acting within _____ seconds after you give an IV bolus.

    60

13. Lidocaine is usually the drug of choice for PVCs. (True/False)

    True

14. Lidocaine will control ventricular arrhythmias about (25/50/75/100)% of the time.

    75

Exercise 31: ADMINISTRATION AND DOSAGE

Study the material in *ICC*, 4th ed., and complete as much of Table 16.4 as you can.

Exercise 32: CONTRAINDICATIONS

1. Mr. Kardiak is on a lidocaine drip for PVCs (we'll cure him or else)—3 mg/min. He develops complete heart block. The danger of continuing lidocaine is _____ _____.

   it might abolish his only pacemaker

2. Administration of lidocaine is dangerous in which of these: SA block/atrial tachycardia/third degree heart block/intraventricular blocks.

   all but atrial tachycardia

3. A patient with severe _____ disease may suffer from a toxic accumulation of lidocaine. Why? _____

   liver
   The liver metabolizes lidocaine

4. Large doses of lidocaine may be hazardous in patients with _____ shock or _____.

   cardiogenic
   pulmonary edema

5. If Mr. Kardiak tells you he's allergic to novocaine and "that stuff they use when they stitch you up," then what?

   Discuss it with the doctor before he has PVCs.

Exercise 33: SIDE EFFECTS

1. The most serious side effect is _____.

   convulsions

2. List six other central nervous system complications

   _____   _____
   _____   _____
   _____   _____

   drowsiness, parasthesias muscle twitching, disorientation agitation, hearing difficulties

3. Watch all lidocaine drips closely, the maximum rate is usually _____ mg/min.

   4

194

DILANTIN

Exercise 34: *USES*

1. In treating PVCs, the doctor will try _____ or _____
   first, and if they fail, _____ may be ordered.

   lidocaine, procainamide
   Dilantin

2. Dilantin may be used to control _____ _____,
   especially when quinidine fails.

   supraventricular tachycardias

3. Arrhythmias caused by _____ toxicity may be treated with
   Dilantin.

   digitalis

4. You are probably more accustomed to using Dilantin to treat _____
   than arrhythmias.

   convulsions or epilepsy

Exercise 35: *ACTIONS*

1. Dilantin (increases/decreases) conduction velocity.

   increases

2. This action occurs in the (atria/ventricles).

   atria

3. Dilantin also tends to (increase/decrease) automaticity.

   decrease

4. ECG changes with Dilantin therapy may include: (widened/no) effect on the QRS
   complex and (lengthened/shortened/no) effect on the PR interval.

   no
   shortened

Exercise 36: *ADMINISTRATION AND DOSAGE*

Study the material in *ICC*, 4th ed., and complete as much of Table 16.3 and Table
16.4 as you can.

Exercise 37: *SIDE EFFECTS: CARDIAC*

1. Because Dilantin _____ automaticity, it could lead to abnormally _____ heart rates.

   decreases
   slow

2. Rarely, Dilantin may cause _____ _____ _____.

   AV heart block

Exercise 38: *SIDE EFFECTS: SYSTEMIC*

1. List central nervous system symptoms associated with Dilantin therapy.

   drowsiness, ataxia, lack of co-
   ordination, nystagmus, nervousness, depression

2. Possible allergic reactions:

   nausea, vomiting, pruritus,
   urticaria, rashes

3. Gingival hypertrophy (swelling of the gums) (is/is not) common on short-term
   Dilantin therapy.

   is not

4. IV administration of Dilantin is by slow infusion. (True/False)

   False

5. Why?

   Dilantin precipitates in solution

6. IV administration is by "bolus" injection. (True/False)

   False

7. Would you believe: injected in the left ear lobe?

   No!

8. Dilantin is given by direct IV but very _____.

   slowly

9. You should inject about _____ mg/min of Dilantin IV.

   50

10. Since Dilantin forms a precipitate, what site on the IV tubing would you use to
    inject the drug?

    nearest to the vein

11. Dilantin IV acts in about _____ seconds.

    15

12. So monitor the _____ closely.

    ECG

13. For what?

14. Also monitor the _____ _____ closely.

15. When giving Dilantin orally, encourage the patient to _____ _____ _____.

16. Why?

	bradycardia, heartblock
	blood pressure
	drink extra water
	minimizes gastric upset

EPINEPHRINE

Exercise 39: *USES*

1. During a cardiac arrest, especially _____ _____, you might expect the doctor to order epinephrine.

ventricular asystole

Exercise 40: *ACTIONS*

Use the information in *ICC*, 4th ed., to complete as much of Table 16.3 as you can. Then try these.

1. Epinephrine is used in cardiac arrest because it stimulates the _____ _____.

pacemaker cells

2. It also (increases/decreases) the heart rate and (strengthens/weakens) myocardial contraction.

increases, strengthens

Exercise 41: *ADMINISTRATION AND DOSAGE*

Study the material in *ICC*, 4th ed., and complete as much of Table 16.4 as you can.

Exercise 42: *CONTRAINDICATIONS*

1. Epinephrine is (less/more) dangerous than Isuprel in treating advanced heart block.

more

2. It can be dangerous for your MI patient because it can increase myocardial _____.

ischemia

Exercise 43: *SIDE EFFECTS*

1. If you have given epinephrine successfully in a cardiac arrest, you must still watch for _____ _____.

ventricular ectopics

2. The patient may experience _____ pain after receiving epinephrine.

anginal

3. Other symptoms you might expect include: _____, _____, and _____.

headache, anxiety sweating

ISOPROTERENOL

Exercise 44: *USES*

1. The most common drug used to treat bradyarrhythmia is _____.

atropine

2. If this fails to increase the heart rate, _____ may be tried.

Isuprel

3. Isuprel should not be used to treat advanced heart block. (True/False)

False

4. Isuprel is best used as an emergency drug until a pacemaker can be inserted. (True/False)

True

Exercise 45: *ACTIONS*

Use the information in *ICC*, 4th ed., to complete as much of Table 16.3 as you can.

1. Isuprel (increases/decreases) automaticity.

increases

2. Isuprel (increases/decreases) heart rate. — increases

3. It (improves/impairs) AV conduction. — improves

Exercise 46: *ADMINISTRATION AND DOSAGE*

Study the material in *ICC*, 4th ed., and complete as much of Table 16.4 as you can.

Exercise 47: *CONTRAINDICATIONS AND SIDE EFFECTS*

1. Isuprel (increases/decreases) the heart's oxygen consumption. — increases

2. Thus, it may be dangerous in acute _____ _____. — myocardial ischemia (infarction)

3. In this situation, the patient may complain of _____ as a result of increased oxygen need. — angina

4. Isuprel may cause _____ _____ or _____ _____ (arrhythmias). — ventricular tachycardia / ventricular fibrillation

5. How? — increased automaticity of ectopic foci

6. Systemic symptoms may include: — sweating, flushing, weakness

7. Central nervous system symptoms are: — nervousness, excitement, tremors, headache, dizziness

8. Isuprel's effect on skeletal and mesenteric vessels is _____. — vasodilitation

9. This can lead to _____ _____ _____. — decreased blood pressure

10. If the monitor shows increasing _____, you'd reduce the rate of Isuprel. — PVCs

11. A syringe of _____ should be at the bedside. — lidocaine

PROPRANOLOL

Exercise 48: *USES*

1. Another name for propranolol is _____. — Inderal

2. In general, propranolol is used to treat which arrhythmias? — supraventricular tachycardias

3. It is used to treat tachyarrhythmias caused by _____ toxicity. — digitalis

4. If lidocaine and Pronestyl fail, Inderal may also be tried in the treatment of _____. — PVCs

Exercise 49: *ACTIONS*

Use the information in *ICC*, 4th ed., to complete as much of Table 16.3 as you can. Then try these.

1. Propranolol (increases/decreases) sympathetic nervous system stimulation. — decreases

2. Propranolol (increases/decreases) automaticity. — decreases

3. It (slows/speeds up) conduction. — slows

4. It (increases/decreases) strength of contraction. — decreases

5. It (increases/decreases) cardiac output. — decreases

6. It is not a drug to be given lightly in patients with acute myocardial infarction. (True/False) — True

Exercise 50: *ADMINISTRATION AND DOSAGE*

Study the material in *ICC*, 4th ed., and complete as much of Table 16.4 as you can.

Exercise 51: *CONTRAINDICATIONS AND SIDE EFFECTS*

1. Because propranolol decreases rate and prolongs AV conduction, it should not be used in _____ or _____ _____.

   bradycardias, heart blocks

2. Because it decreases cardiac output, it should not be used in _____ _____ or _____ _____.

   heart failure, cardiogenic shock

3. Because it affects the lungs adversely, it should not be used in _____ _____ or _____.

   bronchial asthma, bronchospasm

4. Propranolol may cause an excessive (increase/decrease) in heart rate.

   decrease

5. You'd watch the monitor closely for bradycardia and for the development of _____ or _____ _____ _____ _____.

   2nd, 3rd degree heart block

6. You'd check the patient's blood pressure for signs of _____.

   hypotension

7. Respiratory symptoms of _____ or _____ would cause you to discontinue the drug and notify the doctor.

   wheezing, bronchospasm

8. Central nervous system effects might include:

   lassitude, depression

ATROPINE

Exercise 52: *USES*

1. Atropine is given to _____ heart rate.

   increase

2. Thus, it is used in sinus_____, _____ _____, and _____ _____ _____.

   bradycardia, SA arrest slow junctional rhythms

3. It can be used to (increase/decrease) conduction through the AV node.

   increase

4. Thus it may be helpful in _____ and _____ _____ _____ _____.

   1st, 2nd degree heart block

Exercise 53: *ACTIONS*

Use the information in *ICC,* 4th ed., to complete as much of Table 16.3 as you can. Then try these.

1. Atropine (inhibits/enhances) vagal stimulation of the SA and junctional areas.

   inhibits

2. Increased vagal activity (slows/speeds up) the SA node.

   slows

3. When vagal activity decreases, then the _____ nervous system (slows/speed up) the SA node.

   sympathetic speeds up

4. Thus, inhibiting vagal influence allows the SA node to_____ _____.

   speed up

5. Bradycardias due to SA or AV damage (are/are not) speeded up by atropine.

   are not

6. Blood pressure may _____ with atropine.

   increase

7. Cardiac output may _____ with atropine.

   increase

Exercise 54: *ADMINISTRATION AND DOSAGE*

Study the material in *ICC,* 4th ed., and complete as much of Table 16.4 as you can.

Exercise 55: *CONTRAINDICATIONS AND SIDE EFFECTS*

1. Atropine may (increase/decrease) intraocular pressure.

   increase

2. Therefore, patients with _____ should not be given atropine.

   glaucoma

3. For what renal system conditions should atropine be given cautiously?

   urinary obstruction, prostatic hypertrophy

4. In these cases, atropine may cause _____ _____.

   urinary retention

5. For this reason, the patient's _____ _____ should be carefully noted after atropine is given.	urinary output
6. Atropine, less than 0.3 mg or given slowly, may cause _____ _____ of the heart rate.	paradoxical slowing
7. Atropine may also cause _____ _____ heart rate.	excessively rapid
8. Atropine can increase _____ rate more than _____ rate.	atrial, ventricular
9. This can lead to _____ _____.	AV dissociation
10. Rarely, a dangerous result may be _____ _____ or _____ _____.	ventricular tachycardia ventricular fibrillation
11. The monitor should be closely observed for at least _____ minutes after atropine has been administered.	5
12. Systemic symptoms may include:	dry mouth, blurred vision, dilated pupils
13. Central nervous system effects may include:	euphoria, excitability, confusion

DIGOXIN

Exercise 56: *USES*

1. The doctor orders digoxin. Which of the following can you use? digitoxin, Cedilanid, ouabain, digitalis leaf, Lanoxin, digitalis purpurea.	Lanoxin
2. Digitalis preparations are used to control (slow/fast) rate arrhythmias.	fast
3. Digitalis preparations are used especially for (atrial/ventricular) arrhythmias.	atrial

Exercise 57: *ACTIONS*

Use the information in *ICC*, 4th ed., to complete as much of Table 16.3 as you can. Then try these.

1. Digoxin (increases/decreases) myocardial contractility.	increases
2. Digoxin is a vagal (stimulant/blocker).	stimulant
3. Increased vagal stimulation (slows/speeds up) the heart rate.	slows
4. Digoxin also slows the rate of conduction in the _____ _____ and _____ _____ _____.	AV node bundle of His

Exercise 58: *ADMINISTRATION AND DOSAGE*

Study the material in *ICC*, 4th ed., and complete as much of Table 16.4 as you can.

Exercise 59: *CONTRAINDICATIONS*

1. Before the doctor starts Mr. Kardiak on digoxin, he's particularly interested in whether or not you've seen any of the following arrhythmias on the monitor: _____ _____, or _____ or _____ _____ _____ _____.	junction tachycardia, 1st, 2nd degree heart block
2. What lab work should you check before Mr. Kardiak starts on digoxin?	acid-base balance, K, electrolytes

Exercise 60: *SIDE EFFECTS: CARDIAC*

1. Digitalis is one of the safest drugs administered in the CCU. (True/False)	False
2. Digitalis may cause almost any arrhythmia. (True/False)	True

3. List 2 possible arrhythmic side effects of digitalis: | junctional tachycardia, **PAT** with block

4. PVCs caused by digitalis are often in the form of _____. | bigeminy

5. If ECG signs make you suspect digitalis toxicity, what should you do? | Hold the next dose and call the doctor

6. Digitalis should not be given if the heart rate is below _____ without a special order. | 60/minute

7. _____ therapy can decrease the serum _____ (electrolyte) level and thus potentiate digitalis toxicity. | Diuretic, potassium

8. The margin of safety between a therapeutic and a toxic level of digitalis is (small/great). | small

Exercise 61: *SIDE EFFECTS: SYSTEMIC*

1. List the systemic symptoms and signs of digitalis overdose:

   Gastrointestinal system: | anorexia, nausea, vomiting
   Central nervous system: | depression, confusion, lassitude

   Other: | abnormal color perception, blurred vision

2. Compare the usual maintenance doses of:

   digitalis leaf _____ mg | 100

   digoxin _____ mg | 0.25

   digitoxin _____ mg | 0.1

   (Inadvertent substitution of digitalis preparations can be fatal!)

BRETYLIUM TOSYLATE

Exercise 62: *USES*

Look at the monitor. There it goes again: V Tach' or V Fib'. You've given lidocaine, procainamide, and tried defibrillation.

1. For these recurrent or refractory arrhythmias, the doctor may order _____. | bretylium

Exercise 63: *ACTIONS*

Use the information in *ICC*, 4th ed., to complete as much of Table 16.3 as you can. Then try these.

1. Bretylium (blocks/accelerates) sympathetic nervous system discharge at the nerve endings in the heart. | blocks

2. However, first it may cause ventricular _____. | arrhythmias

3. Bretylium (does/does not) reduce myocardial contractility. | does not

Exercise 64: *ADMINISTRATION AND DOSAGE*

Study the material in *ICC*, 4th ed., and complete as much of Table 16.4 as you can. Then try these.

1. In unconscious patients, bretylium is given (diluted/undiluted) until a maximum of _____ mg is given. | undiluted / 30

2. This is done by repeating doses every _____ to _____ minutes. | 15, 30

3. _____ and _____ must both be used before and after the repeated doses.

CPR, defibrillation

4. Why? _____
_____.

There will be no pulse, no oxygenation during this time

5. In conscious patients, bretylium is given (undiluted/diluted).

diluted

6. Bretylium (is /is not) used as a maintenance drug to prevent recurrences.

is

Exercise 65: *CONTRAINDICATIONS AND SIDE EFFECTS*

1. There are no specific contraindications, but bretylium is not used as the_____-
_____ drug.

first-
line

2. At least 50% of the patients receiving bretylium develop _____
_____.

postural
hypotension

3. You'd watch your patient for _____.

lightheadedness, fainting,
vertigo

4. You'd keep the patient in the _____ position and have_____
or _____ ready to give IV.

supine, dopamine
norepinephrine

5. Exactly the opposite, an initial transient _____ may occur.

hypertension

6. An increase in ventricular _____ may also occur.

ectopics

7. Bretylium potentiates the effects of drugs: _____, _____,
_____.

digitalis, dopa-
mine, Levophed

8. Especially dangerous is the use of bretylium with _____.

digitalis

9. Be certain of the mode of administration, it can be _____, _____,
or _____.

bolus, infusion
IM

10. Bretylium is given (diluted/undiluted/both).

both

VERAPAMIL

Exercise 66: *USES*

1. Verapamil is used in (supraventricular/ventricular) arrhythmias.

supraventricular

2. The verapamil on your drug shelf may be labeled _____ or _____.

Calan, Isoptin

Exercise 67: *ACTIONS*

Use the information in *ICC*, 4th ed., to complete as much of Table 16.3 as you can. Then try these.

1. Verapamil is the best example of a new type of drug: _____ _____
_____.

calcium blocking
agents

2. Calcium blockers block the entry of calcium into the _____ _____
thus slowing conduction across the _____ _____.

cardiac cells
AV node

3. It can also slow the rate of the _____.

sinus node or heart

Exercise 68: *ADMINISTRATION AND DOSAGE*

Study the material in *ICC*, 4th ed., and complete as much of Table 16.4 as you can.

Exercise 69: *CONTRAINDICATIONS*

1. Verapamil is contraindicated in ____ _____ or ____ _____ disorders.

AV nodal, SA nodal

2. It should be used cautiously in cases of _____ _____. → congestive heart failure

3. Calcium blockers should not be used with drugs of the _____-_____ type. (Example: propranolol) → beta-blocker

4. You should wait at least _____ hours after stopping propranolol before giving verapamil. → 24

Exercise 70: *SIDE EFFECTS*

1. With verapamil, watch the monitor closely for signs of _____ _____ or _____. → heart block bradycardia

2. Carefully measure the _____ _____ on the monitor strips. → PR intervals

3. You're trying to detect the very first signs of _____ _____. → heart block

4. The most common systemic side effects are _____ and _____. → nausea, constipation

5. _____ may be severe enough to discontinue verapamil. → Constipation

6. Verapamil may potentiate other drugs. Ones to be aware of include: _____, _____, _____ and other antiarrhythmics. → Inderal digitalis, Norpace

POTASSIUM

Exercise 71: *USES*

1. The symbol for potassium is _____. → K

2. This symbol is derived from the word _____. → kalemia

3. Patients with low intracellular K may show _____ (arrhythmia) on the monitor. → PVCs

4. Thus, K administration may sometimes be used to treat _____. → PVCs

5. Digitalis toxicity may cause tachyarrhythmias such as _____ _____ _____ and _____ _____. → PAT with block junctional tachycardia

6. _____ may be used to treat these arrhythmias. → K

Exercise 72: *ACTIONS*

Use the information in *ICC*, 4th ed., to complete as much of Table 16.3 as you can. Then try these.

1. K (increases/decreases) the threshold of excitability. → decreases

2. This would (increase/decrease) the likelihood of ectopic pacemakers. → decrease

Exercise 73: *ADMINISTRATION AND DOSAGE*

Study the material in *ICC*, 4th ed., and complete as much of Table 16.4 as you can.

Exercise 74: *CONTRAINDICATIONS AND SIDE EFFECTS*

1. Patients with _____ problems may have trouble excreting K. → renal

2. If the patient's lab studies show an elevated _____, you'd watch more closely for signs of hyperkalemia. → BUN

3. Normal serum K level is _____ to _____. → 3.8, 5.1 mEq

4. If a patient's serum potassium level is 5.8 mEq, you would (give/withhold) the ordered dose of potassium. → withhold

5. Serum K levels above _____ should be reported, STAT. → 5.1 mEq

6. If your patient's monitor shows _____ or _____ _____ _____, you'd question giving K. | 2nd, 3rd heart block

7. In hyperkalemia you may see increased _____ _____ on the monitor. | AV blocks

8. Any change in rate, rhythm, duration of QRS, should be reported, STAT. (True/False) | True

9. Describe the ECG changes to watch for:
   _____ T wave | narrow, peaked
   _____ QT | shortened
   _____ PR | prolonged

10. Initially, K (increases/decreases) excitability and (increases/decreases) intra-ventricular conduction. | decreases, increases

11. Prolonged IV potassium infusion may reverse this desirable effect. (True/False) | True

12. IV potassium may cause what local symptom? _____ | burning and pain along the vein

13. If this happens, the IV should be (stopped/slowed/left as is). | slowed

14. IV potassium should be diluted in _____ cc of fluid. | 500

15. Flow rate should not exceed _____ mEq/hour. | 20

16. Symptoms of potassium toxicity are: | weakness, heaviness of extremities, listlessness, confusion, drop in blood pressure

17. Oral K may cause: | nausea, vomiting, diarrhea, abdominal pain

NEW ANTIARRHYTHMIC DRUGS: AMIODARONE

Exercise 75

1. Amiodarone may become one of the more popular antiarrhythmic drugs because it does not seem to decrease myocardial _____. | contractility

2. Its effects (do/do not) persist for over a month after discontinuing the therapy. | do

3. It seems to prevent recurring _____ _____. | ventricular fibrillation

4. It (does/does not) slow the heart rate and (does/does not) produce heart block. | does, does

5. Side effects include: corneal _____ and pulmonary _____ and _____. | deposits, fibrosis infiltrates

APRINIDINE

Exercise 76

1. Aprinidine can be used to control most serious _____ arrhythmias. | ventricular

2. Its action resembles that of the drugs _____ or _____. | quinidine procainamide

3. Neurological side effects you must watch for include: _____, _____, _____ _____, and _____. | tremor, ataxia double vision, nervousness

4. These side effects (may/may not) limit its use. | may

203

ENCAINIDE

Exercise 77

1. Encainide seems to be effective in treating _____ ectopics.

   ventricular

2. You'd watch the monitor for increasing _____ _____ and widening _____.

   PR interval
   QRS

3. You'd also watch the patient for signs and symptoms of _____ _____ _____.

   congestive
   heart failure

FLECAINIDE

Exercise 78

1. Flecainide has the advantages of effectiveness against a wide range of _____, a (short/prolonged) effect, and relative safety.

   arrhythmias, prolonged

2. However, it can cause complete _____ _____ or _____.

   heart block, aystole

3. Thus you'd watch the monitor for prolonged _____ and _____ intervals.

   PR, QRS

4. Flecainide would probably not be used for patients with advanced_____ _____ or cardiogenic shock.

   heart
   failure

MEXILITENE

Exercise 79

1. Mexilitene can be considered as similar to an "oral _____".

   lidocaine

2. Its use (is/is not) limited by adverse side effects.

   is

3. Systemic side effects to watch for include: _____, _____, _____, _____, and _____.

   tremors, nystagmus
   dizziness, ataxia, confusion

4. Mexilitene (can/can not) be used in combination with other drugs to reduce its side effects.

   can

TOCAINIDE

Exercise 80

1. Tocainide also resembles an "oral _____".

   lidocaine

2. Its side effects (are/are not) mild.

   are

3. It (can/can not) be used on a long term prophylactic basis.

   can

Table 16.3. Drug Action Chart

	Direct Action					Indirect Action				
Drug	Automa-ticity	Excita-bility	Conduc-tivity	Myocard-ial Cells	Contrac-tility	Cardiac Output	Vagal/ Sympath.	Heart Rate	Conduc-tivity	Contrac-tion Force	Comments
Quinidine											
Procain-amide											
Norpace											
Lidocaine											
Dilantin											
Epine-phrine											
Isopro-terenol											
Propran-olol											
Atropine											

↑ = increase
↓ = decrease
⌀ = no effect

Table 16.3. Drug Action Chart (cont'd.)

| Drug | Direct Action | | | | | Indirect Action | | | | Comments |
	Automaticity	Excitability	Conductivity	Myocardial Cells Contractility	Cardiac Output	Vagal/ Sympath.	Heart Rate	Conductivity	Contraction Force	
Digoxin										
Bretylium										
Verapamil										
Potassium										

Table 16.4. Drug Administration and Dosage Chart

Drug	Mode	Dosages			Action Time	Blood Level		Warnings	Comments
		Loading	Repeat	Maintenance	Prophylactic		Desired	Toxic		
Quinidine										
Procaina-mide										
Norpace										
Lidocaine										
Dilantin										

Table 16.4. Drug Administration and Dosage Chart (cont'd.)

Drug	Mode	Dosages				Action Time	Blood Level		Warnings	Comments
		Loading	Repeat	Maintenance	Prophylactic		Desired	Toxic		
Epine-phrine										
Isopro-terenol										
Proprano-lol										
Atropine										

Table 16.4. Drug Administration and Dosage Chart (cont'd.)

Drug	Mode	Loading	Repeat	Maintenance	Prophylactic	Action Time	Desired	Toxic	Warnings	Comments
				Dosages			Blood Level			
Digoxin										
Bretylium tosylate										
Verapamil										
Potassium										

209

Answers to Table 16.3. Drug Action Chart

Drug	Direct Action						Indirect Action				Comments
	Automaticity	Excitability	Conductivity	Myocardial Cells	Contractility	Cardiac Output	Vagal/Sympath.	Heart Rate	Conductivity	Contraction Force	
Quinidine	↓	↓ (esp. Atrial)	↓ (esp. A.V. node)	depress	↓	↓	Vagal block	↑	↓		Vagal effect can counteract direct
Procainamide	↓	↓	↓	depress	↓		Vagal block	↑			Can cause A.V. or I.V. blocks
Norpace	↓		↓				Vagal block		↑		Vagal effect can ↑ V. response
Lidocaine	↓ His-Purkinje	↑ ventricle Ø Atria	Ø blocks		Ø	Ø					
Dilantin	↓ SA and ectopic		↑ Atrial								Avoid in S.A. arrest or bradycardias
Epinephrine							↑ Sym.	↑		↑	Lg. doses = ↑BP, ↑peripheral resistance
Isoproterenol	↑		↑ A.V.	↑ O₂ need			Sympath. stimulant	↑		↑	Caution in coronary ischemia
Propranolol	↓		↓ Atria and His		↓	↓	Sympath. block				
Atropine					↑		Vagal block	↑	↑		Allows sympath. control

210

Answers to Table 16.3. Drug Action Chart (cont'd.)

Drug	Direct Action					Indirect Action					Comments
	Automaticity	Excitability	Conductivity	Myocardial Cells	Contractility	Cardiac Output	Vagal/Sympath.	Heart Rate	Conductivity	Contraction Force	
Digoxin	↑		↓ A.V. and His		↑		Vagal stimulant				Caution in H.B. ↑ ectopics
Bretylium					φ		Sym. blocker				↓ BP Initially, causes v. arrhythmias. Restores S. rhythm
Verapamil			↓ A.V. node ↓ SA node	Ca blocker				↓			Do not use in AV or SA nodal disorders, or with beta-blockers
Potassium			↑ A.V. and I.V.								

Answers to Table 16.4. Drug Administration and Dosage Chart

Drug	Mode	Dosages				Action Time	Blood Level		Warnings	Comments
		Loading	Repeat	Maintenance	Prophylactic		Desired	Toxic		
Quinidine	p.o.	300 mg	q 3 h × 3	200-600 mg q 6 h	200-300 mg q 6 h	begins in 2-4 h	5-7 mg/L.	→ 8 mg/L.	Wide QRS AV block	Do not exceed 1.6 g daily without serum quinidine levels
Procaina-mide	IV (2 g in 500 ml.) IM— p.o.—	100 mg (25 ml.) 500 1 g	q 5 min. do not exceed 1 g/h	2-4 mg. or 1 g/6 h for 24 h					Causes hypotension	Stop if QRS widens 50%, PR increases, or 1st or 2nd H.B. occurs.
Norpace	p.o.	300 mg	150 mg q 6 h			2 h lasts 6 h			Watch for: CHF, V. Tach., Urinary retention, Constipation, Dry mouth, Blurred vision.	Contraindications: Heart failure, Renal disease, Urinary retention, Hepatic disease, Glaucoma
Lidocaine	IV IM (rarely)—	50-100 mg or 1 mg/kg body weight 200 mg—	q 5 min. up to 300 mg/h q 5-10 min.	1-4 mg/min. Mix: 3 g of 2% in 500 ml = 6 mg/ml	D.C. when arrhythmia ceases	60 seconds, bolus lasts 15 min.			Caution in liver disease.	Contraindications: 3rd H.B., advanced A.V. or IV blocks; Large doses in cardiogenic shock or pulmonary edema.
Dilantin	IV slow push p.o.	125-250 mg at 50 mg/min. 200 mg	q 15 min. if needed 100 mg q 6 h	do not exceed 750 mg/h 100 mg tid	begins in 15 sec., maximum 5 min.				Do not mix in IV—precipitates	

Table 16.4. Drug Administration and Dosage Chart (cont'd.)

| Drug | Mode | Dosages | | | | Action Time | Blood Level | | Warnings | Comments |
		Loading	Repeat	Maintenance	Prophylactic		Desired	Toxic		
Epineph-rine	Subcu'	0.1-0.5 mg								Caution in angina or MI—may increase ischemia.
	IV	0.25-0.5 mg	2-8 mcg/min.							
	Intra-cardiac	5-10 cc of 1:10,000								Intracardiac in arrests only.
Isopro-terenol	IV—mix 1 mg in 250 ml, 1 cc = 4 mcg	2.4 mcg/min.	up to 6-10 mcg/min.						Can cause V. Tach. or V. Fib.	Use micro-drip
	Intracardiac or IV for vent. stand-still	.02-0.1 mg								
	IM or subq.	0.1-0.4 mg	q 2-4 h			begins 15-30 min.				
	Sublingual	10-20 mg	q 3 h							
Atropine	IV bolus	0.3-1 mg	in 5 min.	Can repeat in 4 h. Do not exceed total 4 mg		begins 1-3 min., lasts 4 h				
Proprano-lol	IV slow push	1-2 mg/min.	5 min. then do not repeat for 4 h			begins in minutes, lasts 3 h			Watch for: hypo-tension, heart failure	Contraindications: H.B., CHF, asthma
	p.o.				10-30 mg q 4-6 h					

Table 16.4. Drug Administration and Dosage Chart (cont'd.)

Drug	Mode	Dosages				Action Time	Blood Level		Warnings	Comments
		Loading	Repeat	Maintenance	Prophylactic		Desired	Toxic		
Digoxin	IV	25 mg	0.25 mg in 3-6 h, then decrease	total 24 h not to exceed 1.2 mg		begins in 15 min, maximum 1 h			Toxicity causes any arrhythmia, especially bigeminy.	Contraindications: 1st or 2nd H.B. Acidosis, alkalosis, hypokalemia increase sensitivity to digitalis.
	p.o.	0.5 mg	0.25 mg q 6 h × 2 to total of 1.5 mg	0.125 mg 0.25 mg daily		begins in 2-6 h				
Bretylium tosylate	IV undiluted	5 mg/kg	10 mg/kg q 15-30 min 30 mg total						Unconscious pts only in V Fib.	Use CPR & defibrillation
	IV-mix 500 mg in 50 cc	5-10 mg/kg over 10 min.		1-2 mg/min IV mix or 5-10 mg/kg q 6 h						Not a first-line treatment.
	IM	5-10 mg/kg	q 2 h prn							
Verapamil	IV	5-15 mg over 1-2 min.				1-5 min.				For PAT 80% successful
	p.o.	80 mg or 120 mg qid								To slow vent response in A. Fib.
Potassium	IV slow drip	40 mEq in 500 ml, slowly 2-3 h							Never bolus	Contraindications: renal insufficiency, 2-3 H.B. Check serum levels.
	p.o.		40-80 mEq daily in divided doses							Mix oral in fruit juice, give with full glass water.